Jewish Paths toward Healing and Wholeness

Jewish Paths toward Healing and Wholeness

A Personal Guide to Dealing with Suffering

Rabbi Kerry M. Olitzky
Foreword by Debbie Friedman

For People of All Faiths, All Backgrounds
JEWISH LIGHTS Publishing
Woodstock, Vermont

Jewish Paths toward Healing and Wholeness: A Personal Guide to Dealing with Suffering

© 2000 by Kerry M. Olitzky

Permission to reprint material from the following sources is gratefully acknowledged:
Prayer for healing from *On the Doorposts of Your House* reprinted by permission of the Central Conference of American Rabbis.
Asher yatzar (p. 99) and *Refa na lah* (p. 105) reprinted by permission of Congregation Sha'ar Zahav, San Francisco, California.
Selection from *When the Body Hurts, the Soul Still Longs to Sing* compiled by Rabbi Nancy Flam from a collection written by her students. Reprinted by permission of Rabbi Nancy Flam.
"Mi Sheberakh" from *And You Shall Be a Blessing,* music by Debbie Friedman, lyrics by Debbie Friedman and Drorah Setel, © 1988 by Deborah Lynn Friedman (ASCAP). Reprinted by permission of Sounds Write Productions, Inc. (ASCAP).
"You Are the One (Reb Nachman's Prayer)" from *Renewal of Spirit,* music by Debbie Friedman, lyrics by Debbie Friedman (based on Reb Nachman's prayer), © 1995 by Deborah Lynn Friedman (ASCAP). Reprinted by permission of Sounds Write Productions, Inc. (ASCAP).
Selections from *The Book of Words: Talking Spiritual Life, Living Spiritual Talk* by Lawrence Kushner © 1993, *Soul Judaism: Dancing with God into a New Era* by Rabbi Wayne Dosick © 1997, and *Healing of Soul, Healing of Body: Spiritual Leaders Unfold the Strength & Solace in Psalms* edited by Rabbi Simkha Y. Weintraub © 1994 reprinted by permission of Jewish Lights Publishing.
Prayers by Rabbi Rami M. Shapiro reprinted by permission of Rabbi Rami M. Shapiro.
"When I Am Lonely" by Danny Siegel, The Town House Press, Putaboro, North Carolina, 1999, reprinted by permission of Danny Siegel.

Library of Congress Cataloging-in-Publication Data
Olitzky, Kerry M.
Jewish paths toward healing and wholeness : a personal guide to dealing with suffering / Kerry M. Olitzky.
p.   cm.
Includes bibliographical references.
ISBN 1-58023-068-7 (pbk.)
1. Healing—Religious aspects—Judaism.
2. Suffering—Religious aspects—Judaism. 3. Spiritual healing. I. Title.
BM538.H43 045 2000
296.7—dc21   00-009365

10   9   8   7   6   5   4   3   2   1
Manufactured in the United States of America
Cover design by Drena Fagen
Text design by Sans Serif, Inc.

Published by Jewish Lights Publishing
A Division of LongHill Partners, Inc.
Sunset Farm Offices, Route 4, P.O. Box 237
Woodstock, VT 05091
Tel: (802) 457-4000   Fax: (802) 457-4004
www.jewishlights.com

"Jewish healing is a discovery and rereading of Jewish texts, a reinterpretation and invention of Jewish rituals developed through the eyes and heart of one who has experienced loss. All lead to bringing a compassionate presence to Jews who are ill, grieving or despairing, to their families and their caregivers."

—*Rabbi Rachel Cowan*

B'yado afkid ruchi, be'eit ishan v'a-ira, v'im ruchi gevi-a-ti, Adonai li v'lo ira.
Into God's hands I entrust my spirit, when I sleep and when I wake;
and with my spirit and my body also, as long as God is with me, I will not fear.

—Adon Olam, *from the liturgy*

Dedicated to
David Nathan Meyerson, *z"l*

May his memory be a blessing to us all.

Contents

APPENDIXES

Acknowledgments

There are many people who helped my family and me find the Jewish path to healing. They have all become our teachers. In particular, I mention and thank those individuals who helped me immeasurably throughout the development of this manuscript in ways that they may not even be aware of: Rabbi Daniel Brenner, Dr. Daniel Einhorn, Rabbi Peter Knobel, Dr. Carol Ochs, Dan Schechter, Rabbi Elliot Stevens, Rabbi Robyn Tsesarsky, and Marvin Zauderer. I am indebted to Sharon Gutman who shared her story of struggle and survival with me before the idea for this book had even been articulated. I also recognize the labor of Dr. Mark Straus, an early collaborator in this endeavor when the book was to take a different shape and form.

Similarly, I want to acknowledge the good works of these organizations that are engaged in a variety of healing projects and shared their materials with me—their ideas are implicit in much of what I have written: Central Conference of Reform Rabbis; CLAL: National Jewish Center for Learning and Leadership; and Synagogue 2000. I must also single out the National Center for Jewish Healing (and its subsidiary, New York Jewish Healing Center), which has been doing groundbreaking work in the field. By name, I mention Susie Kessler, Aaron Lever, Janet Sherman, and Rabbi Simkha Weintraub, without whose assistance this work would not be possible. I am mindful of the profound influence this evolving grassroots organization has had on the entire field of healing in the Jewish community, so it is difficult to determine the extent or specificity of its influence on these pages. Ahead of time, I apologize if I have inadvertently used an idea or even a word without properly acknowledging its original source as the National Center for Jewish Healing or one of its staff members.

I must also acknowledge the groundbreaking work of Rabbi Yoel Kahn, formerly at Congregation Shaar Zahav in San Francisco, who laid the groundwork for services of healing. His own *"Shema Koleinu:* A Liturgy for Healing" (prepared with Rabbi Nancy Flam) significantly informed the section on healing services in this book.

There are no words available to thank my editors, Elisheva Urbas and Lisa Yanofsky, whose keen insights kept me on course when I might have gone astray. They constantly asked the right questions and were there with just the right amount of guidance. While the words and ideas are mine, they both share in the blessing of this book and the work of healing that it assists people in doing. And to my publishers and friends Stuart and Antoinette Matlins, I offer my humblest appreciation. They constantly challenge me to reach deeper and higher at the same time, standing by me as we journey together through the desert.

I must also thank my new colleagues at the Jewish Outreach Institute, Dr. Egon Mayer and Nastaran Afari, who provide the constancy of collegial support in the form of a "team" that makes such work possible, as well as the members of the board, with the indefatigable Terry Elkes as its president. They have helped me easily make the transition from one community to another, constantly reminding me of the blessing inherent in the work we do.

Finally, I would like to express my gratitude to the many students who have given me the privilege of sharing these ideas with them in the classroom, in the hospital, and in brief moments of encounter. They have helped me to learn anew each day of God's miracles.

Most people will argue that responsible scholars and writers do not reveal the names of their sources when preparing a volume for public consumption. That is true. However, many of the people whose stories appear in these pages are witnesses to the miracle of healing. Many want their names attached to their stories and want their stories told, so I share most of the stories of healing in their own names, with their permission, relating them in their own voices. I am simply their spokesperson. I acknowledge their candor and willingness to share with me and with you.

My family has helped me to understand the journey of healing that we embarked on together. To Sheryl, my soul's partner, and to our boys, Avi and Jesse, who constantly provide me with unconditional love, the greatest ingredient for healing.

—Rabbi Kerry (Shia) Olitzky

Foreword

◈

Debbie Friedman

I have been engaged in the process of healing for all my adult life. Once faced with the physical limitations imposed upon me, I found that the healing process took on new dimensions. It was no longer enough to intellectually acknowledge the constant struggle in which I was engaged. My challenge was different now. I had to move beyond my seeking out a place in the world which was safe and comfortable. This was war, and at this time I was forced to take part in what was to be a constant battle with my body. I often had no choice but to surrender to the power of its constraints.

I knew that the only way to survive this torture was to transcend it. My body had to become a metaphor for something in our lives that would make sense. Within this nightmare, my life, I had to find a world of hope and promise.

It was the prayer *Asher yatzar* that first awakened me to the possibility of finding meaning in my life in the face of my newfound "enemy." Not everything was working according to the divine plan which God had created. Sometimes it was impossible to stand before God and pray because there was so much not working. But after some time, I came to see that what worked, worked. This, too, was a part of God's wisdom, and for this I could be grateful. I knew too that even if I could not find my place in the

Asher yatzar prayer, I could always turn to the prayer *Elohai ne-shama* in which we are uplifted by the concept of God giving us a pure soul; a soul created by God, formed by God and breathed into us by God.

This is the prayer to which I run when my body has given way. This is the place I go when I have done too much and I am unable to function. I am always hopeful that something good and helpful will come to be as a result of such an episode. I ask myself, "What I can learn from this experience? What is my body telling me? How can I make this experience my lover, my friend and partner on this unpredictable and bumpy road toward meaning and understanding?"

How can I find ways to embrace this monster when what I really want to do is vacate, throw in the towel and cry out in anger: "Okay, you win, now let me out of my misery." I remember lying immobilized. Was it I who stood up to Goliath? Certainly, I could not entertain the possibility of the "valley of the shadow of death." I had hoped that goodness and mercy would follow me all the days of my life and that I would "live in God's house forever."

And sometimes *that* was all I needed: a reminder that my ancestors held these prayers and poems and writings close to their hearts in times of celebration and in times of need. We who read this book, *Jewish Paths toward Healing and Wholeness,* seek out the same hints of hope as those who came before us. This searching is what has sustained us through time and what sustains us now.

Jewish Paths toward Healing and Wholeness provides us with the resources that reinforce our spiritual and emotional lives. By becoming more tolerant and understanding of ourselves and our respective afflictions, and by learning to see ourselves as the victors and not the victims, our afflictions will become our teachers, our friends and our partners in life and in prayer. The "process of healing" will ultimately become the "promise of healing." We begin

that healing in our immediate world, but the effects resonate beyond in our partnerships with one another and God. These are the
seeds of *tikkun olam*. This is the Jewish path toward healing and
wholeness.

Debbie Friedman is an internationally renowned composer, liturgist, teacher
and performer.

Introduction

✺

Healing Is Possible

Through a relationship with God bolstered by the application of Jewish sacred texts and supported through an exploration of the self, we can find healing. I believe it and I will help you explore that belief too. That's probably the main reason why you have opened up this book, and it's why you are willing to enter into a dialogue with me and with the many others whose stories of healing fill these pages.

Prior to reading this book, your only hope for the possibility of healing probably came from the world of traditional medicine. As a result of your illness—or the illness of someone you love—scenes of hospitals, medical laboratories, treatment centers, and physicians' offices have become familiar sights. The medical routines have become commonplace. We measure our days by the endless hours of waiting. We're overwhelmed: intimate questions posed by strangers; people poking and touching; invasive tests of all kinds; complicated machinery of cold ceramic and steel with electronic brains that whirl, beep, and buzz.

We may have previously considered it unimaginable, but we have actually gotten used to this persistent assault on our senses and our selves. In an ironic sort of way, the familiarity of these hectic places that are home to the marvels of medical science provides us with some comfort at this turbulent time in our lives. They provide us with promise and direction. The routine gives us security. From a medical perspective, it's all part of the conventional path toward a cure. Some physicians refer to it as "normal protocol." We're told that it is all necessary for our eventual well-being. So we endure it all and focus our attention on it, rarely daring to question, afraid that it might undermine our care. We simply do whatever we are told until we become weary from our interaction with the world of traditional health care. Then we are ready to gain some balanced perspective on our illness, ready to embrace a message of hope through a more spiritually based healing process. And it is exactly this path to healing that this book promises to explore.

Healing Is Not the Same as Curing

Spiritual healing is decidedly different than a physical cure. Some imagine them as one and the same. Others argue that one clouds over the essence of the other. For many of us, they are inseparably linked. Many people I counsel understand that it is nearly impossible to get to a physical cure without first building a foundation of spiritual healing—that's why they come to me for guidance and direction. Yet the spiritual process of healing is so interwoven with disease and physicality that they may seem indistinguishable. This is probably the primary reason why so many people can't seem to see the difference, or worse, why they discard one in favor of the other. Maybe they even reject the possibility of spiritual healing out of hand.

When the processes work seamlessly together to spiritually heal *and* physically cure, when spiritual healing helps forge a path toward a physical cure, it is an astounding and overt transformative phenomenon. While we don't see the intricacies of the process, we literally feel reborn. It is not unlike air travel. When everything works out correctly, we board a plane in one city and get off in another at the appointed time. Aside from an occasional bump or two, we may have no idea what it really took to get there. We take for granted all the efforts of so many people that made it possible for us to get from one place to another safely and comfortably, especially the pilots. Just like plane rides that aren't always so smooth and efficient, as much as we wish it was different, the process of health and healing does not always work out that way either. To fully understand this path we are taking toward well-being, we must distinguish spiritual healing from physical cure. Unfortunately, it is sometimes only when we are ready to die, when the physical disease has overwhelmed the body even though the spirit seems fully healed, that we can understand the necessary distinctions that have to be made. And then, though not physically cured, we may be fully healed.

Suffering and Pain

What can be said about the relationship between spiritual healing and physical cure can likewise be said about the relationship between suffering and pain. Spiritual suffering must be differentiated from physical pain, although they too are intertwined so closely that it's nearly impossible to distinguish one from the other. We suffer spiritually when we do not grow from our illness, when we do not learn from the experience of physical pain. This recognition may not make the pain any less real, but it can reduce—and potentially eliminate—the suffering that is associated with it. Rabbi Levi Yitzchak of Berditchev, an eighteenth-century Hasidic rabbi who became well-known for his challenges to God's actions, was overheard to say during one of his more reflective moments, "Eternal presence of the universe, I am not asking You to show me the secret of Your ways, for it would be too much for me. But I am asking You to show me one thing: What is the meaning of the suffering that I presently endure? What does it require of me? What are You trying to tell me through it? I do not mind that I suffer, let me only know that it is for Your sake." Like most of us, this sage wanted to know that his suffering had meaning. Once he discovered that it did, his suffering abated. That's the logic of a spiritual approach to healing.

Through disease we can learn so much about our inner spiritual life that some may be motivated to say that it is *almost* worth bearing the burden of the disease to discover it, as long as we can be guaranteed that we will survive. One cancer survivor told me that had she not developed the disease, she would not be the person she is today. She might not have seen herself so clearly in the divine light that was radiated in her new relationship with God, and she could not imagine learning the profound lessons she learned in any other way. So, as difficult as it might seem right now, you have to find the means to welcome your disease and embrace it like you would a teacher from your childhood whom you only now realize influenced your life so intensely. Somehow you have to find a way to reach inside yourself and open up to the disease. It is part of who you are and what you can become.

In my own family, I am convinced that my wife and I are different people today than we were before her cancer. Our relationship is stronger than we might have ever imagined in the romance of our youth. In struggling with her illness, I know that we both transcended many crises, especially the midlife crisis, the remnants of which continue to plague so many of our peers even after they have moved through this stage of their lives. We just refused to let it enter the gates of our home.

We learned from this experience that before you can embrace spiritual healing, you have to be willing to accept the disease and call it your own, a frightening proposition. People are simply afraid of doing it. Who wants to make a personal claim to a serious illness? Why would we want to intentionally identify with it and name it as part of who we are? After all, we are now fighting with our very lives to rid ourselves of it. Many would rather call it "other," estrange themselves from it, just as the biblical book of Leviticus seems to speak of *tza'arat* (a disease that is usually interpreted as leprosy but probably refers to a variety of physical and spiritual diseases). The people of the Bible did not want to speak of such diseases, and people still don't want to talk about them today. Such conversation would force them to admit that they are sick, that they carry a disease, that they may be contagious. But the patient must take control of the disease so that it does not control him or her. If you feel that the disease is defeating you, that you cannot take hold of it, then healing of any sort may soon be out of reach to you. So grab on with all of the inner strength you can muster, and if you need help, then invite your friends and family to join you in the effort.

The Torah provides a model to help underscore this point. It reminds us that all who struggle with illness resemble the biblical patriarch Jacob who wrestled with God. According to the book of Genesis, on Jacob's journey toward reconciliation with his brother Esau, whom he tricked out of his birthright and blessing, Jacob decided to rest for the night. In a natural response to a long journey, Jacob realized that he needed to gather his strength to face the difficult task ahead of him. The travel had been long and arduous and he was exhausted. Although he longed to reunite with his estranged brother, Jacob was also anxious and fearful. As a precaution, he even separated his family into two camps to protect them. When we recall the story of the struggle of this biblical ancestor with the unknown in the middle of the night—and the Torah is ambiguous about many of the details of this struggle—we sometimes forget that Jacob, who emerged with the new name of Israel after his encounter with God, arose wounded. He walked away limping.

Though he survived victoriously, Jacob carried a constant reminder of his encounter with the other side. But in the midst of the struggle, perhaps as a result of it, Jacob opened himself up to a relationship with the Divine. Did he wrestle with an angel, a heavenly being who served as a messenger of God? Or was it simply a confrontation with the dark side of his inner self? The answer is not apparent after reading the biblical story or from the commentary made by the generations of rabbis and scholars who have explicated it. That Jacob struggled throughout the night is the only thing that is evident. Anyone who has spent a night in fitful sleep can relate to Jacob. In the logic of the spiritual world, however, it is clear that in Jacob's woundedness he became whole. Jacob had to endure the physical pain of the struggle with the darkness and its result, but his spiritual suffering was over. This is the lesson that illness can conceivably impart—that however intense and unrelenting, physical pain can yield spiritual healing.

What Is Healing?

Healing is both a journey and destination. It is both process and the result of that process. I frequently hear people say, as they are recovering from illness or surgery that is relevant to it, "I am healing" or "I am healed." In either case, some people read the words "spiritual healing" and immediately translate it as "physical cure." For many, they will indeed be the same, for as the body becomes well, the spirit may also become whole. But physical cure may be all that matters to them. Like many of us who are seeking easily accessible answers to the ultimate questions of life, these readers will look to this volume for a step-by-step, how-to guide that will provide specific directions for achieving a physical cure. When they do not find such directions here, they may leave these pages disappointed and perhaps search out medical professionals to "fix" whatever part of them is "broken." For others, such a physical cure may not yet be on the horizon of research and discovery. Regardless of our state of "dis-ease," to be cured of bodily illness, one must find the path of healing of soul. Without it, even a physical cure may not be fully possible. That's why this book is not specifically concerned with medical care.

However, there should be no misunderstanding about the indispensable role of physicians and other medical personnel on the Jewish path to healing. This is a joint endeavor in which many parties should be involved, each one supporting the work of the others, each one providing a context in which the efforts of the others are most effective. Those who are responsible for seeking a physical cure must join together with those who are working toward spiritual healing.

We will learn that progression toward spiritual healing is not about being cured from a physical illness. In fact, many people, such as Rabbi Nancy Flam who regularly works with those seeking healing, believe that we don't even have to be ill to achieve spiritual healing. Instead, this route is a foundation for spiritual living in which a physical cure may also be found. It is about seeking wholeness in our lives, for in that wholeness, spiritual healing can emerge. This idea stems from the Hebrew spiritual construct of *shelemut,* translated as "wholeness" and directly related to the word *shalom,* a word usually translated as "peace." It is illness that makes us feel broken and threatens to keep us that way. But we don't have to allow it, and we do have the capacity to change it. The spiritual healing that can come from physical illness can put us on the passage toward wholeness—*shelemut*—for it is often the illness alone that prompts us to seek healing. This book will help show you how. Within its pages, it offers each of us the chance to be fully restored to a state of spiritual healing, of *shalom.*

How Do We Seek and Find Healing?

Before we can find the path to healing, we have to acknowledge our illness and embrace it as part of the inner life of the self, part of the spiritual dimension of our lives. Our illness is more than just an objective disease that afflicts the body or the mind; it has become part of who we are. As difficult as it is to do, begin by acknowledging forthrightly that all that is happening is real even though it sometimes seems like we are merely acting out a role in someone else's life. We think, "This can't be happening to me. This is not my life." We may feel like we are living in a fog; our former life, the daily routine of yesterday, becomes a distant blur. It is as if the world around us has stopped spinning or we have just lost interest in whirling with it since illness entered our lives.

I vividly remember going into the New York City subway one particular morning, rushing with the crowd as part of my daily commute from the suburbs. It started out as a seemingly typical day. Then this idea struck me—on the way to my office, fighting to retain my place on the train among hundreds of people, I thought to myself, "I am surrounded by all these people and they have no idea what I am going through, the burden of knowing that the one I love is ill." The realization nearly paralyzed me. I was busy just living my life, doing what I thought I was supposed to do, when it all happened. Life was not supposed to work this way, not for me, not for us. But it did, and on that day I made a commitment to myself and to God that we were going to find our way through it. I knew then as I do now that we could find our way toward healing and be healed as a result.

Once we have acknowledged our illness and our relationship to it, we have to get certain obstacles out of the way. Most of us confront the same barriers to recovery although they sometimes occur in different orders. Neither unique nor surprising, these hurdles must be overcome. We move them out of our way by grabbing hold of them. Although I could make a list of them for those who would hope to skip directly to the issue of cure, I must emphasize that the process of healing demands that we individually identify and then overcome each impediment on our own. Otherwise, I would be robbing people of the spiritual insights that emerge from confrontation with these obstacles.

Our initial and natural impulse is to deny disease or its severity. We play it down. We don't tell our friends. We may even choose to keep it from some members of our family. As an expression of our concern for others, we don't want to alarm people. Perhaps we are afraid that if we share the severity of our disease with others it will make them uncomfortable. And some, in fact, will keep their distance once they learn of our illness. It is a hard lesson we learn about the stuff of which people are made, including our friends. But denial does not lead anywhere and it certainly does not lead toward healing.

As soon as we are diagnosed with a disease, we want to deal with it and be done with it. The surgeon may advise us that "cutting it out" will mean the end of it. When my wife was first diagnosed with cancer, the doctor said that surgery would take care of it and then we wouldn't have to be bothered with it for the rest of our lives. We believed him, until the cancer returned five years later, which taught us a new lesson: serious illness is a chronic life condition that forces us to be ever-vigilant. Every sniffle or common virus gives us pause. The first question we ask the physician is always, "Is the cancer back?" Even with his assurances, we always carry a measure of doubt with us.

Everyone wants to be fully cured from a disease. When we are seriously ill, we are prepared to do whatever is needed to be done and then get on with our lives. If you can be cured and don't have to deal with the disease again, that's great. A broken bone heals and the broken area often comes back even stronger than before. The body places a patch around the bone that eventually gets smoothed out, especially in younger people. There is hardly any evidence of the original break. But when we survive any significant trauma, like a life-threatening disease, it remains with us forever, even when it is no longer a physical worry.

When I counsel people who are seeking a divorce, they are all in a hurry. Once they have made the decision, they just want "it" to be behind them as quickly as possible. Gently, I advise them that divorce is forever, particularly when there are children involved. They can never fully put it behind them. And for those who struggle with alcoholism, drug dependency, or other compulsive behaviors, they are always "in recovery," whether their sobriety is recent or not. Survivors of the Holocaust, who think they have put that horrible part of their lives behind them, realize, particularly as they advance in years and their bodies remind them of their past, that they can never be fully free of the traumas they once experienced. The collection of these experiences contributes to who we are. Moreover, in the best sense of the word, these experiences may be the root cause of the new self that has emerged, of the person we have become.

Why Me?

"Why me?" we may ask. "Why am I the one who is sick?" There are probably no satisfying answers although we will consider some of the classic Jewish responses in chapter 1. Even if we were to find an answer, it would make the disease no less real, no less virulent. Why waste so much energy on these questions? Because the quest for answers, the very asking of the questions, can help us negotiate a path toward healing. And there are lots of questions that come up, often when we least expect them.

The unrelenting, multilayered question of "Why?" rages a fierce battle deep in the recesses of the soul, so it has to be addressed. If it is not, it threatens to eclipse everything else in our healing process. But we may mistakenly think that if we find a satisfying answer to this query, it will provide some measure of comfort and relief. The scientific community has socialized us this way. Everyone wants the graphic details and specific descriptions, deluding themselves into believing that this line of questioning will offer relief. But it just isn't so.

At the beginning of our journey toward healing, there are questions that demand our immediate attention. Often, they arise so fast that we can't keep up with them. What is the extent of the disease? What is the preferred method for treatment? How serious is it? How long have I had it? What caused it? What could I have done to prevent it? Is it genetic? Will I pass it on to my children? How long will the treatment take? When can I go back to work? What should I tell my family? And then the inevitable question, the one that goes right to the essence of our very being: *Why did it happen to me?* Or the question that perplexes the person sitting alongside in the doctor's office, waiting impatiently for the exam to be concluded or the tests to be over: *Why did it happen to the one that I love?* As caring individuals, the essential question is: *Why does it happen to anybody?*

Some people, regardless of the strength of connection to their Jewish roots, will look to Judaism for answers, thinking that rabbinic theology, whether ancient or modern, will provide a set of explanations for their disease. In this book, we will learn that although rabbinic teachings can't remove the obstacles to healing, we still have to explore them. Our faith demands it. When some rabbis propose the theory that physical illness is simply a punishment for sin, the specific transgression of God's commandments, many contemporary Jews find it difficult to comprehend this interpretation of life despite being socialized in this school of thought. We dismiss it out of hand. Yet, such explanations give us pause. They nag at us even though many who are sick will eventually reject all of them.

I infer a different interpretation of the classic instruction that comes from the rabbis of the Talmud who wrote, "when a person sees suffering come upon him, he should examine his [we would add: her] ways" (Babylonian Talmud, *Berakhot* 5a). We don't deserve the disease. No theological explanation will convince me otherwise. But we may have contributed to its emergence. That's how I've come to understand this lesson. That's why we have to start work on our spiritual lives immediately. Some of our behaviors need to be changed; by devoting our attention to them, we can overcome the obstacles that are blocking our way to healing. We might want to examine past behaviors and link them to our illness. As we look to changing them, we can begin to build a foundation for the future.

As we contemplate these ideas, plenty of deep-seated anger may surface along with the question of "Why?" And the anger is complemented by a sense of helplessness, of feeling alone. These reactions, particularly anger, can potentially suppress our immune systems when we do not confront them and root them out. Thus, without the spiritual process of healing the anger, we will not be able to sustain a physical cure.

When he initially learned about his leukemia, my colleague Rabbi Hirshel Jaffe wrote in his diary/autobiography, eventually published as *Why Me? Why Anyone?*, that he was not angry at first. Ironically, it was not until he was on his way toward being cured that he got angry. By that point, Rabbi Jaffe could work a little, but he could not return to the hectic daily routine that had formed the foundation of his life's work. That's what got him angry. It may seem odd that he was well on the road toward physical well-being before anger welled up in his soul. But that's the point: These feelings do not come in a predictable order or for the same reasons. Anger can arise at any time and because of anything, including feelings of injustice or inadequate explanations to our questions. In this case, it was the anger that helped Rabbi Jaffe

jump-start the spiritual healing process even after he was physically cured, and that's what made it essential. He faced it, held on
to it for the purpose of examination, and then let it go.

Focusing on Healing Instead of Explanations

As a practitioner rather than a theologian, I believe that most of
our theological questions have to be set aside so we can focus on
healing and the best path to take. That's what I had to do. When
we first learned of my wife's cancer, it came as a shock. No one
expected it, not even our family physician. My wife was young,
healthy, watched what she ate, and got regular exercise. Like most
of us, she worked too hard, trying to raise a family and make a living. Among the many reactions I had to the harsh news presented
to us by a rather stoic surgeon was a somewhat self-centered response; I inwardly focused on my own questions rather than on
hers. I wondered: "Perhaps it was something that *I* did!" I was
worried that my life of faith had failed our family. Would my belief in a benevolent God stand up to this test? What could I really
do to help heal her? I may have led countless people in prayer, but
I had previously paid inadequate attention to its power over individual lives. My wife's illness motivated me to reconsider what
faith, belief, and prayer had to offer the sick. The eventual renewal
of my faith is woven into the fabric of this book. It might even be
the impetus for writing it.

Similarly, our friend Debbie, who struggles with an illness
that continues to baffle her physicians, taught me that healing is a
continuous process, just as any serious illness is chronic, even if the
doctors don't categorize it as such. She lives with a chronic illness
and is constantly struggling to free herself from it. Debbie asked
"Why?" in between the spirit-lifting notes of her musical compo-
sitions, and out of her pain came music that brings healing to herself and others.

Spiritual healing comes through the process of reaching the Divine. Through this process, we are able to redirect the negative energy that results from the physical disease and make it positive. There are several mechanisms that can provide us with road markers along the way: ritual, Jewish texts, and prayer. Like Jewish tradition, this book is rich with them. Rituals moor us in the drifting seas caused by a physical disease. The application of Jewish texts offers the primary touchstone for spiritual healing. Prayer is about attempting to initiate a dialogue with the Divine. It's like saying, "Hey God, I'd like to talk to you," but adding "please" just to be polite and a bit humble. The traditional form makes it easier to dial God's number, so to speak.

All readers have specific needs, which this book seeks to address. Whether as someone who is seriously ill or as one who loves someone who is fighting a disease, together we face the illness. And I join you in your struggle, as does God, although you may not feel God's presence in your life right now. That's why traditional Judaism recommends the development of a ritual life that is contextualized with regular prayer.

For many, the first Yom Kippur after learning about an illness can be overwhelming. Sue, an older friend whose deteriorating pulmonary disease increasingly steals her lifebreath from her, told me that the words of the ancient *unataneh tokef* prayer cut deeply into her for the first time in her life after being diagnosed, although she had faced death many times as a childhood survivor of the Holocaust. The tears flowed freely as the words of this old, familiar prayer seemed to stick in her throat. When she mouthed the words, it was as if she was bringing them into being: "Who shall die by fire and who by water? Who by illness and disease? Who by suffering?" She held these words engraved in the prayer book alongside the numbers invisibly tattooed on her arm, and they gave her a renewed directive for her life. She heard them repeatedly throughout her Yom Kippur day in prayer: Repentance *(teshuvah)*, prayer *(tefillah)*, and charity *(tzedakah)* can mitigate the severity of the decree. She knew what she had to do, what she had learned early in her life: *Teshuvah, tefillah,* and *tzedakah.* As she approached the open ark that year, she was nearly brought to her knees, humbled in the presence of the sacred, totally drained by the journey that she was just beginning. She had found her course to healing.

Finding the Individual Path

Each reader has individual needs. It is admittedly difficult to meet them all in the pages of one book, but there is one thing we share in common: We all face illness—if not of self, then someone in our family needs God's help, and needs our help. We yearn to bring them healing.

There is not one family I know that has not faced the ravages of illness and disease. Age, which used to be the measuring stick for major disease, has become irrelevant. Cancer, in particular, seems ever present. Women and men are equally threatened. The list is endless. And some doctors believe that potential cancer cells are present in everyone's body. Our immune system is constantly fighting them off until one day, it is no longer able to stave off these destructive cells and illness strikes. We can combat this unfortunate reality by making ourselves whole once again.

Rabbi Rachel Cowan teaches us that "Jewish healing affirms that our tradition can speak with wisdom to the condition of brokenness, that it can illuminate our path when we are in the depths and calling out for help. It teaches that the metaphor for *shelemut,* wholeness, is a cracked vessel. When we are struggling to make our way on this path, a Jewish approach to healing steadies us with texts, with community, with *niggunim,* and with silence. Above all it comforts us with the knowledge that Jews have walked this path for thousands of years, finding light in the midst of darkness. It teaches us that we are not alone. Our soul may be downcast, but we can yet hope in *Adonai*."

This is a book about personal belief in the form of spiritual healing, the necessary first step that must be taken before the body can also be healed. It is based on my experiences, academic, communal, and personal. For those who are skeptical, leave your incredulity and Cartesian doubt outside of these pages—if only for the time it takes to read them. You can always pick them back up after you have finished reading, should you still find it necessary to do so. Come join me on the journey toward healing as we enter into the gateway of the spirit in prayer, community, and in a renewed relationship with God.

ONE

✠

A Healing God

I believe in God. I believe in a God who heals as part of a divine expression of love. I believe in a God who heals as part of the relationship between the Divine and the human. It is important to make statements of belief at the outset so that this belief cannot be taken for granted, for it emerges from the depths of my soul. It fills my entire being with optimism and light. It is this optimism that brings healing and eclipses the potential for suffering. Like Moses' spontaneous prayer for his sister's health in the Torah after she is stricken unexpectedly with some unknown illness (*El na, refa na lah;* O God, heal her please), this simple statement reverberates throughout my daily routine, even as its echoes can be heard throughout history in the lives of other individuals.

Like you, I have many doubts and plenty of questions regarding God, particularly at times of illness and misfortune. I consider this uncertainty to be an important part of my struggle with faith. Faith is not about simple belief; it is a complex dimension of our humanity that is filled with inner conflict. As part of an exploration of God as healer, we also have to consider the relationship of suffering to the Divine, a question that unfolds at the same time. But this belief in God informs what I can affirm about God's role in healing. It is this struggle that has guided my exploration of what may be called a *theology of healing,* and therefore provides a spiritual map for this chapter. Alongside relationships with family and friends, the one you have with God is the primary relationship that must be considered in the context of the Jewish path toward healing. For the person who believes in God, regardless of the specific dimensions of that belief, ultimate faith in God is indispensable to healing.

When facing illness, you may not feel like considering words scripted by thinkers and teachers who make their homes in the academy. You may even find it difficult to concentrate on reading. There are so many things on your mind demanding your attention that reading may seem like an additional burden you are reluctant to take on. But reading this book will help, as will thinking about the ideas it explores. Take the time you need to read *and* reflect.

This is indeed the right time to explore your belief in a God of healing. Illness forces us to consider issues about God we have avoided during our lives. At the same time, our vulnerability during illness brings us closer to God in uncanny ways that are similar to how we might feel about God during the High Holy Days and different from how we feel the rest of the year.

This chapter provides a historical development of ideas and also follows my real experience with them—an approach that reflects a pattern created out of the encounters with God and healing that most people have. These are ideas I was forced to confront as a student of Torah and as one who was forced to learn new Torah during my wife's illness. Many of my views may have originated in the classroom, but more than anything else, they are concepts that evolved out of my own experiences and those of others as they sought healing for themselves or for those they love.

This is not an overly technical chapter about Jewish theology because discussions at this early juncture should not be rife with scholarly jargon. But it is important to lay bare the foundation of belief as key to Jewish healing. Even though we may only want guidance and direction, it is important to speak from the perspective of our experience, and then to provide a context for that conversation within the framework of Jewish intellectual thought. We cannot avoid entering into a dialogue with our tradition and what has been said about God and healing throughout the long history of our people. It is that dialogue that becomes part of the historical tradition as we, too, enter into it.

This discussion might be too academic for some, particularly for those who seek only practical resources, which can be found throughout the later chapters of this book. For those who prefer the cerebral to the utilitarian, the conversation may seem insufficiently intellectual. However, in an exclusively intellectual discourse, you run the risk of avoiding the emotional, profoundly human dimension of the conversation. After all, we yearn for healing and want to figure out how to access it as efficiently as possible. As such, in addition to providing a basic theological framework, this chapter talks primarily about the path toward faith and belief in God as a healer and what seems to be most relevant when illness enters your life.

Historical and Contemporary Perspectives

The early rabbis, perhaps more than any other collective group of clergy before the modern period, lived among the people and experienced daily life with them. Their work continues to serve as a model for us all. When I was a rabbinical student still early in my studies, I was asked to visit a young woman at a local hospital who was struggling with life-threatening cancer. While I was waiting to see her, as a means of gaining some clarity and direction for the task ahead, I studied the rabbinic debate concerning a particular prayer, specifically regarding the progression it followed before it was secured a place in the formal liturgy. It was a prayer that I might be moved to pray with an ill patient. At the same time, I questioned the relevance of my study of liturgy and the discussion of the rabbis. How meaningful was their discussion if it gave me no insight into how to bring comfort and healing to this young mother who was fighting for her life? But my study—the words of the rabbis sensitively crafted into prayer—did offer me profound insight. I recognized then as I do now that the debates of the rabbis have their place in our conversation about healing. These Jewish thinkers faced the limits of human life and so this chapter includes the perspectives of the scholars in our tradition, as well as those ideas that emerged directly from my interactions with many people who have wrestled with the concept of God as healer versus God as an entity that condones suffering. Some of these interactions are reframed by Jewish thought, beginning with classic Jewish theology and followed by contemporary responses. In later chapters, I will provide a variety of resources that will enable you to put many of the ideas that are discussed in this chapter into practice.

Does God Punish the Wicked for Their Deeds?

I was raised with a rather traditional concept of reward and punishment. I suspect that most people were, particularly if they attended a synagogue school in North America. This idea was constantly reiterated by my parents and teachers, often unknowingly. Thus, it was the first thing that I can remember thinking about as I confronted these same ideas as an adult. The Torah, which records the spiritual journey of our people through history, is quite clear about reward and punishment, particularly as the rabbis interpret the text for us: The righteous are rewarded for their good work and the wicked are punished for their wrongdoing. Even if this idea presents an intellectual struggle for us—we want to believe it but we have trouble doing so—most of us conduct our lives in ways that reflect this sentiment. Sometimes it comes as a knee-jerk reaction to our children's misbehavior or to some un-kindness done to us. However it manifests, we communicate things through our behaviors that clearly reflect our belief in a system of reward and punishment that is often beyond our comprehension.

The prophets also read this message of the Torah in order to emphasize it for us. It is repeated in one form or another through-out biblical literature by a variety of personalities. Isaiah said it most effectively when he wrote: "Tell the righteous it shall be well with them, for they shall eat the fruit of their deeds. Woe to the wicked, it shall be ill with them, for what their hands have done shall be done to them" (Isaiah 3:10–11). There is no doubt that Isaiah believed that all Israel would be rewarded for their right-eous behavior and punished for their wicked deeds. As a result, this became an essential ingredient of his message to the people.

The psalmists, as historical poets laureate of the ancient Jewish people, saw it the same way. In the ninety-second psalm, one of the psalms we read each Friday evening as we make the transition from the workday world to Shabbat, we acknowledge God's role in the system of reward and punishment. As part of the introduction to the Shabbat worship service, we recite it as a com-munity, and emphasize this doctrine by singing these lines to-gether aloud:

> But they [the evil doers] will be destroyed forever. . . .
> The righteous will flourish like a palm tree,
> And grow mighty like a cedar in Lebanon. . . .
> To declare that God is upright,
> My rock in whom there is no unrighteousness.
>
> *(from Psalm 92)*

I'm convinced that most of us would be satisfied were the wicked punished and the righteous rewarded in this straightforward way because we believe that *we* would be counted among the righteous. Perhaps if it is too presumptuous to call ourselves "righteous," certainly few among us would be willing to refer to ourselves as "wicked." Indeed, even those of us who have doubts about this world view still often try to apply it to the world we see. How often do we hear a story about someone apparently undeserving of suffering who seems to be punished continually? Too many of us are aware of people in our community who have been through a period of bad times (loss of job, perhaps a divorce, or the tragic death of someone they love) only to find themselves now struggling with a serious illness. Some will call it bad luck, others will try to rationalize it some other way. But there will be some who are courageous enough to ask the profound question (usually spoken to onself), "What did he (or she, or I) do to deserve all this?" The rabbis of the Talmud considered the same question and advised: "When a person sees suffering come upon him [we would add: her], he should examine his ways" (Babylonian Talmud, *Berakhot* 5a). We may never discover a reason for our suffering, but we have to be unafraid to search for it, even outside traditional parameters.

Searching for Answers

As a rabbi, I often visit sick people in the hospital or in their homes. My visits usually elicit profound theological questions that emerge as a result of illness. Some patients see me as a representative or spokesperson of God. They have questions for God and, therefore, they expect me to be able to answer them. Some only want answers that affirm their ways of thinking. Others are looking for a theological framework in which to understand their illness. At first, I was taken aback by the perspective that illness is a direct result of our behavior, meted out by God. How could I be God's delegate? Then I began to realize that I am—like others— a channel for bringing God's presence into the life of someone who is ill. I believe that we are all potential outlets for God's voice to be heard in the world. This is an awesome challenge and responsibility, and it is very humbling, but, in fact, I have become God's messenger of sorts—a responsibility that we all share. It is one of the things that prompted me to write this book. I want to help people get at the root of perplexing theological questions like, *Did I do something to deserve this?* and *How can I find healing for myself and others?*

The real problem with the answers to these questions lies with our perception of self. Perhaps it would be better to classify actions rather than people, so we can determine whether the action is punished or rewarded rather than the people who do them. In this framework, there are no wicked or righteous people, and the world is not painted in black and white. Instead, there are people who sometimes do evil things and people who sometimes do righteous deeds, but few who may be considered thoroughly righteous or completely wicked, especially with those who live among us. Most of us live in a world in between the two. It's what some like to refer to as being "good enough." But despite how we have lived our lives—or perhaps as a direct result of it—illness comes to teach all of us how to change the manner in which we live, regardless of how good we think we are.

Illness can teach profound lessons about life and our relationships with others if we are willing to listen to the disease. Jeff and Susan, congregants whom I worked with early in my rabbinate, learned the lesson early in their marriage. They were young parents whose baby—their first child—was born with a life-threatening disease. Suddenly realizing that they were anticipating a lifetime of care for her, they were not angry, nor did they ask God why their innocent newborn daughter was born with such a birth defect. Instead, they wanted me to help them understand the lesson that God wanted them to learn through their baby's life and their relationship with her. They believed that their daughter had come into the world for a reason and was in need of loving and caring parents. Years later when I saw them again, I realized that I had never seen such an outpouring of love between parents and child. I felt that they were indeed the ones divinely chosen to care for this special child. They confirmed for me Viktor Frankl's assertion that humanity's essential drive is to create meaning. Jeff and Susan gave meaning to their child's illness.

This approach will not satisfy everyone. Perhaps that is why the rabbis came along and modified the equation of reward and punishment somewhat from what the Bible specifically taught. They sought an explanation for what they experienced in their own lives. They saw that the righteous often went unrewarded while those who did evil went unpunished. By introducing the notion of "the next world" (the afterlife), they suggested that reward and punishment are not restricted to this world. Instead, when considering the balance of good and evil in the world, we must look at this world and the next. Maybe this is why we say the psalm mentioned above on Shabbat—as a taste of the redemption that the righteous will find in the next world. But this is still not an adequate explanation for many people. As a result, some contemporary rabbis have sought to address the issues that they deemed unsatisfactorily answered by their predecessors, while still pursuing the role of God as healer.

The Theory of a Limited God

Like many children, when I was a child I thought that God was capable of doing anything. It is what my parents taught me, and this idea was reinforced by my own rabbi and those teachers who tried to direct my early religious education. After all, I learned early that God created the world and all that is in it. In our daily service of prayer, we recited: "How great are all Your works, *Adonai*. In wisdom You created them all." And each year, we re-learned the story of Noah in the book of Genesis, and how the world moved from paradise to corruption, all as a result of the ac-tions of humans. It seems as though God had no choice but to de-stroy the world and everything and everyone in it. So I thought, as I was repeatedly taught to believe, that God would reward me for my good behaviors and punish me for doing things that were not so good, even those pre-adolescent behaviors of which my parents and teachers were ostensibly unaware. I reasoned: If God could destroy the entire world, God could easily get rid of me. While this notion was easy to accept when I was young, it became increasingly difficult to affirm as I moved into a long-lasting re-bellious adolescence and beyond.

I began to cast this story together with others I had heard. If my parents and teachers taught me this particular idea that ap-peared untrue, then many other things they taught me must also be false. Along with other members of my peer group, I rejected most of the traditional values of my childhood and did not revisit them until adulthood. Yet the idea that God would punish me for what I was doing continued to unnerve me because I realized that some of those teenage pranks might have actually been deserving of punishment. And I knew in the depth of my soul—an area I was just on the brink of discovering—that there was more to this question of punishment.

When my mom developed cancer while I was in Israel studying at the age of sixteen, I was totally overwhelmed by the news. It was not merely that the disease threatened to take her from us as it had brutally taken my grandfather, who was an in-tractable giant in my eyes; that would have been hard enough to accept. What really troubled me was that I wondered what she did to deserve the disease. I knew her to be a good person who had worked hard and provided my brothers and me with a foundation of Jewish values with which to navigate the world. Perhaps it was even one of the ingredients that eventually put me on a spiritual course for life. On reflection, I agonized over whether it was something that my brothers or I had done that caused her disease.

Rabbi Harold Kushner answered these questions for many of us years later in 1981, the same year I was ordained a rabbi. In his bestseller, *When Bad Things Happen to Good People,* he shared his personal story with us: As a rabbi, he struggled with faith as he watched his young child suffer and eventually die from progeria, a disease of premature aging. During his early professional life, he had set aside many of his doubts as he was ministering to his congregation. But that wrenching experience finally helped him understand what God is and is not capable of doing, regardless of what we may ask of the Divine. His understanding offered him great release from the responsibility he might have otherwise felt about his son's disease. Moreover, it showed millions of people that rabbis also have difficult questions about God. Rabbi Kushner's words gave many others permission to rethink the classic notion of an omnipotent God as the only possibility. As a result of his pursuit to find the answer to one of life's most difficult questions— Why do the good seem to suffer?—Rabbi Kushner helped an entire generation heal. Further, Rabbi Kushner claimed that, rather than undermining his faith, his new outlook strengthened him and renewed his belief in a benevolent and healing God.

In his book, Rabbi Kushner takes on the classic Jewish theology of the Bible and of the rabbis and offers us a bold, alternative approach. In answering this question, he challenges the traditional understanding of God that most of us learned through our studies with Hebrew scriptures, often aided by traditional commentary. Taking to task the model that is perpetuated by a classic understanding of the Bible, Kushner suggests that the concept of God is irrelevant to supernatural intervention. In his read of Jewish history, this kind of intervention is not the paradigm that has been suggested by the experience of our ancestors. Instead, borrowing a theme from one stream of rabbinic thinking, Rabbi Kushner suggests that God is only able to suffer along with us, which God has done with the Jewish people throughout history, and concludes that God cannot do anything to change events in the everyday world.

Nevertheless, he notes that we can gain profound solace from God in the very midst of our suffering in ways that we cannot achieve from even the most empathic of humans. Rabbi Kushner writes: "We don't need to beg or bribe God to give us strength or hope or patience. We need only turn to the One, admit that we can't do this on our own, and understand that bravely bearing up under long term illness is one of the most human, and one of the most godly, things we can ever do. One of the things that constantly reassures me that God is real, and not just an idea that religious leaders make up, is the fact that people who pray for strength, hope and courage so often find resources of strength, hope and courage that they did not have before they prayed." The notion that God suffers along with us and consoles us, regardless of whether or not we choose to accept the theological consequences of Rabbi Kushner's thinking, is, in itself, healing. For the first time in our study of Jewish sources, we are given license to believe in a compassionate and benevolent God who may not be able to directly cure the sick, but who heals us nonetheless.

Rabbi Kushner presents a persuasive argument for what he calls a limited God. It is a statement that some label as audacious, even blasphemous. How does a human being deign to place limits on the Almighty when the limitations may be a result of our restricted human view on the world? The classic Kushner challenge goes something like this: If God is good and if God is allpowerful, then there should be no evil in the world; since there is indeed evil, and we have all experienced it, then God must either not be good or God must not be all-powerful. Many of us relate to Kushner's position, because we have all experienced what appears to be the limitations of God.

I have felt the reality of divine limitation in my work as a rabbi even when I have not articulated it in the language of Jewish theology. When I have stood at people's bedsides and prayed for their health, too often I have found that my prayers went unanswered and that the illnesses did not abate. As a result, I would ask myself: "Did my personal behavior undermine the efficacy of my prayers? Were they not answered because I failed?" Or perhaps, "Was the person for whom I was praying not brought back to health as result of something he or she did?" Yet I have also known occasions when God answered my prayers directly, causing sickness to recede and disease to be cured. I firmly believe that my wife's cancer is continually held in abeyance as a result of my prayers and those of our family and others who care deeply for her. So I make sure that I continue to pray for her health with each of my daily prayers—and our sons and others in our family do the same. This belief in the power of prayer informs my rabbinate and my religious life.

Prayer: Placing Your Existence in God's Presence

I began to lead a large suburban congregation at about the same time that Rabbi Kushner's book was published. Having just concluded my formal seminary training, it was at the beginning of my religious journey as a rabbi. As soon as I arrived, my congregants asked me to preach about Rabbi Kushner's position. They were intrigued by it. His book had made the *New York Times* bestseller list and everyone was reading it. They wanted my opinion. I really think that most of them just wanted me to affirm Rabbi Kushner's position because it was consistent with their own perspectives on

the world. I knew that if I did so—whatever conclusions I drew—
my words would impact on the rhythm of the entire congregation and reverberate throughout the entire Jewish community.
Among my congregants there were also those who wanted me to
disarm Rabbi Kushner and, as a religious scholar, dismantle his argument. They feared, as I did at the time, that Rabbi Kushner was
undermining the foundation of classic Jewish theology, the basis
on which the Torah, as the touchstone for Jewish spirituality, is
built.

Though my congregants were liberals raised with a rational
approach to Judaism, some still clung inwardly to a belief in a God
that responds to prayer and intervenes in the world to heal those
who suffer. This attitude about traditional values frequently surfaced, particularly when there was a death in the community. On
some level, my congregants literally believed the words of the
daily prayers for healing that are included in the *Amidah,* the core
prayer in Jewish worship. So they yearned for a metarational understanding of Judaism and healing.

I refused their request to take on Kushner in public. I could
not argue religious philosophy with this colleague from the pul-
pit. As I saw it, it was not really the theology that was at the heart
of his book or in healing. I had learned through my own experience with life and death that there are many things more important than a well-developed articulation of a particular theology.
Kushner wrote of his own reason for writing the book, ". . . out
of my own need to put into words some of the important things
I have come to believe and know." The writing of this book
brought him comfort, the same solace that it did for millions of
others. I could not challenge a grieving man as he tried to raise
himself above his pain. Through this transformative act of spiritual
leadership, he invited others who had suffered to join him in his
journey back to wholeness. He brought healing to his pained soul
through the writing of the book and the helping of others.

Kushner's work reminded me of the familiar rabbinic refrain: Words that come from the heart enter the heart.

My colleague Rabbi Steven Moss, who is a chaplain at Memorial Hospital Sloan Kettering in New York, expressed my own quandary: "I recall once being asked to pray psalms for a seven-year-old boy who was in a coma. As I prayed the ancient words, I knew I was not sure of the reason I was praying. Was I asking for the child to come out of the coma and live a vegetable-like existence? Was I praying that the child would miraculously awaken from the coma and be totally cured of cancer? Or was I petitioning God to mercifully take this child's life? In truth, I was asking for all three, as well as for none at all. For, by this act of prayer, I was not saying to God that I wanted one solution over the others; for each, in real-life terms, had its own difficulty. By this act of prayer, I was doing the only thing I knew to do at this desperate moment, which was to place this boy's existence in God's presence, through my presence of love and care for this child."[1]

Nature Is without Morality

Rabbi Harold Schulweis, spiritual leader of Valley Beth Shalom in Encino, California, addresses the same question as Rabbi Kushner, but reaches a different conclusion. Schulweis believes that God and nature are not the same. Instead, he maintains that our only option is to classify nature and its implications as *chol,* secular, and morally neutral, separate from God. This approach frees us from the inclination to defend God for each natural disaster or personal illness, and it does not place limits on God, as Kushner would have it. Rabbi Schulweis' approach posits that nature is neither hostile nor unfriendly to the moral universe, but rather is totally irrelevant to it. Here he echoes the words of the rabbis, "The world pursues its natural course and stolen seed sprouts as luxuriantly as seed honestly acquired" (Babylonian Talmud, *Avodah Zarah* 54b).

For if we believe that the world is all God, then we are not able to separate anything from it, even nature, which may be considered God's creation. Even if we argue that it is not the same as God—for those who believe in God as the Creator of the universe, who created nature and set the laws of nature into motion even if unprepared to intervene in them once they have been established—then nature may still be considered of God.

I believe that God is indeed separate from nature. Nevertheless, God can be discovered in nature, as humans act to transform nature to consecrated ends. Thus we must make sure that if we embrace Rabbi Schulweis' approach, we work to bring sanctity to all of our efforts in healing, including prayer.

A Theology of Balance

For those among us who clearly see God *in* nature, Schulweis' explanation helps us with one aspect of our struggle, but leaves us with other problems to resolve. He is not the first to look for some sort of a balanced approach in theology. Like other philosophers of his generation, the great medieval theologian/physician Moses Maimonides often wrote about the pursuit of the golden mean (or what I like to call the "golden middle"), the midpoint between two extremes, as a means of establishing balance in life. In the 1960s, it is what people liked to call "centering," a spiritual place that you strive toward. Maimonides believed that for a life to be soulful, it cannot be lived in the extremes. Instead, individuals must find their place halfway between any given set of polarities.

Rabbi Nancy Flam, a pioneer in this nascent field of healing, has applied this notion of a golden mean in her attempt to come to grips with a theology of healing. Out of her years of experience working within the healing community, she has frequently seen the direct manifestation of this theology. Acknowledging the two opposing attributes of God, typically labeled as *din* (usually translated as "justice") and *rachamim* (usually translated as "mercy" or "compassion"), she suggests that the idea of *din* is misunderstood. Instead of the harsh imposition of judgment, which the rabbis suggest reflects the *din* side of God, Flam understands *din* to refer to the amoral imposition of limits. Like nature, limits have no relationship to morality. Illness and disease emerge within the limits of the physical world, and they can thereby be understood as coming directly from God as the creator of the physical world with its laws and its limits. It is precisely what the philosopher Cordovero suggests is inherent in things, because they have to remain within their own boundaries. Thus, *tziduk hadin*, the statement ("Blessed is the Righteous Judge") that Jewish tradition requires upon hearing bad news (particularly a death), is an affirmation of this idea.

While illness is an expression of God's attribute of judgment *(midat hadin)*, according to Rabbi Flam, healing is an expression of God's attribute of mercy *(midat harachamim)*. This *rachamim* (from the Hebrew word for "womb" and reflecting similar aspects of creation) makes it possible for us to live within the reality of *din* (judgment). It is the Jewish impulse to add *rachamim* so that it overcomes *din*. According to the Talmud, God is reputed to pray, "May it be my will that my mercy *[rachamim]* may prevail over my other attributes" (*Berakhot* 7a). By seeing the potential balance of *din* and *rachamim* in our lives, we may be better able to recognize God at all times, especially in the context of our illness.

God Helps Those Who Help Themselves

Perhaps Rabbi Flam sees this pursuit of *rachamim,* or healing, as a means of the individual to help oneself. We know from Jewish literary history how important it is for Jews to help themselves. It is a core value, just like helping one another. With the help of insightful writers of midrash, there are those who are persuaded that God unsuccessfully initiated the creation of the world and, disappointed with what was created, subsequently destroyed it. After numerous failed attempts, God remade this world with the human species as co-creators.

The responsibility of these co-creators is to complete the process of creation that God started. Similarly, God can initiate the healing process but needs humans to help move it toward completion. Many people think that this idea refers only to medical personnel, and see medical science as the source of all modern miracles. However, as we have learned from research and personal experience, the individual has to be willing to help him- or herself on the road to recovery. When physical healing does not take place, some may draw the conclusion that the individual was unwilling to help him- or herself, but that is not the case. Spiritual healing transcends the body (even though there can be no separation of body and soul in Judaism) and can be pursued by anyone with a resolve to reach for *rachamim*.

What We Cannot Comprehend

In my work in pastoral care and counseling, I have been witness to incredible feats by those who sought healing. It is the responsibility of a rabbi to share intimate moments with a variety of people, including congregants, students, associates, and friends. I have been privileged to be with people at various stages of their lives, struggling with them through their pain and suffering, while also humbled by the feat of their recovery. Early in my career, I vividly remember being awakened in the middle of the night by our family physician who also happened to be a congregant. Groggily, I answered the telephone. There had been a fatal traffic accident involving the son of a family in my congregation and his friend. A drunk driver lost control of his car on a rural road at the Connecticut shore and took the lives of these two young men. I dressed quickly and drove over to the home of my congregants. Both families were there. While only one was Jewish, I ministered to both of them that evening and over the weeks and months that followed. Amidst their grief, the Catholic family exhibited a certain peaceful resignation. They were convinced that for some unfathomable reason, God had chosen to invite their son to "return to him," and were even wistful about his journey to a better place. The Jewish family begged me to explain, longing for resolute comfort in their pain. They wanted to believe that God had a plan for their son—which included his young and untimely death—but they just could not do so.

Rabbi Lawrence Kushner, one of the leading spiritual teachers in the Reform movement and author of numerous books on mysticism, offers this insight to explain their struggle: "In moments of heightened awareness, we often are overcome with the sensation that everything is happening according to a plan. We have merely raised ourselves to a level from which we can comprehend part of the bigger picture. We cannot see the whole thing, but for a moment we discern larger pieces and, above all, our intended place within the whole. And, even more surprising, at such times of 'rising to our destiny,' we actually feel a heightened sense of freedom. We are 'free' to be what Heaven has intended us to be or not, but we are not free to be something else."[2]

There is much that we cannot comprehend about God or the plan God has for all of us. Some scholars believe that God is beyond human understanding so that any attempt to try to understand God or even reach God is presumptuous. The psalmist said it best in the beginning of the ninety-second psalm:

How great are Your deeds, *Adonai*
Your thoughts are elusively profound.
The ignorant cannot fathom them,
Nor does the fool understand them.

The Book of Job

God was as inscrutable for the characters who struggled with the Divine in the Bible as God remains for us. Elsewhere in the Bible, not far from the book of Psalms, we find the classic tale of suffering in the form of the book of Job. As the Bible describes Job, he seems too perfect to be real. Job is an all-around good guy. He is a model father, husband, and community member. In our own day, while we know people who are good, decent people, there are few, if any, who even approximate the goodness of Job, who is described in glowing terms. This serves to strengthen the message. It appears that God is actually bragging about Job's goodness. In response, Satan argues, "Of course Job is faithful to you. You shower blessings on him. Should you take these blessings from him, let's see how faithful he might be."

God accepts Satan's challenge at Job's expense, afflicting Job with boils, destroying his home and cattle, and killing his children. Job's wife urges him to give up his faith. In the original story as scholars understand it, Job refuses to give up his faith at his friends' urging and is properly rewarded for his steadfast belief. In the biblical account that we have, however, which early Jewish editors may have modified from earlier folk literature, Job confronts God and Job's friends espouse the traditional position of faith: God rewards the faith of the righteous. Job wants to know why he was punished and his friends tell him that it is a presumptuous request. He wants to know what his children did to deserve their deaths and claims that he had tried to live decently. Job's friends lash out at Job and tell him that he has fooled them, feigning religious belief only when things were going well. Thus, he is deserving of the punishment. Eventually, God appears in the context of a whirlwind to reply to Job. While God's position is hard to understand, Job eventually becomes silent, realizing he has said too much to God.

The story of Job illustrates the theological paradox of unexplained suffering with one addition: We learn at the outset that Job is a good person, undeserving of punishment. We know that Job's friends are wrong when they suggest that Job must really deserve his punishment. If they took an alternative position, they would have to argue that God is malevolent because the book of Job presupposes God as all-powerful. Job simply resigns himself to living in an unfair world because there is no mediation with regard to God. He believes that God is beyond comprehension, rather than being malevolent. Many of us have chosen to resign ourselves to that position as well. Yet, the idea of prayer or contrition as a mechanism that can influence divine decision suggests that mitigation with regard to God is indeed possible. Nevertheless, the message that emerges from the classic story of Job is confirmed in our everyday life: God is unknowable and beyond our human ability to understand.

Trusting a God Who Is Beyond Our Understanding

Rabbi Lawrence Kushner suggests that we only need to understand one thing about God: "God puts you where God needs you. You are where you are *supposed* to be. The job you are doing may not be easier on account of this, indeed it may be harder, even more urgent, but now you are centered, focused, clear. So this is where I am supposed to be. I always thought I was supposed to be somewhere else, doing something else, being someone else. But I realize now that I was mistaken. This does not mean that I can't or will not be doing something else. Just right now, I am where God wants me."[3]

It sounds like a truism, but there are indeed some things, particularly in the life of the spirit, that are just beyond our understanding. We may come to understand these issues one day or at least gain some measure of comprehension. But there is one reality that, as humans, we will never come to fully understand: That is God. Cynics may ask, "What is the function of God?" But that is like asking, "Why is there love?" When we make a decision to live a life reflective of the covenant forged at Sinai, the notion that God is beyond our understanding can be liberating. We don't understand why things happen the way they do. But somehow we have to develop the strength of faith that allows us to place ourselves in God's hands without any regret.

The Paradox of Living

Trying to find a theology of healing that makes sense in the postmodern world presents us with a paradox. While science informs much of how we navigate the world today, we have come to understand its shortcomings. Instead, we learn that religion is more helpful in unraveling the mysteries of the world. Among other things, we have learned that the questions we ask are often more important than the answers that science provides. It seems to be part of the human condition to be simultaneously rational and metarational. Thus, our beliefs about God and healing should be constructed along a progressive continuum that reflects the various stages of our suffering and our faith. We experience different facets of God as we move through our lives, and our belief in God changes as we progress through these experiences. Similarly, we confront different aspects of God as healer as we move forward on our path toward healing. Thus, our theology of healing changes as well. Our journey is dynamic. As a result, so is our theology. There are times in which we keenly feel the power of God's healing presence. It may overwhelm us, filling us with awe and dread. At other times, God seems distant and remote. It appears as though God is disinterested in the world and disconnected from our individual human lives. In part, this sense of alienation and estrangement is a dividend of living at this juncture in history, which challenges us with the paradox in the first place.

The philosopher/theologian Martin Buber argued that evil may be defined as the absence of relationship and direction in our lives. Since the model for all of our relationships should reflect the one we establish with God, we can potentially combat the evil of suffering by developing relations with each other and with God. Such a process will help us recognize that we are never alone: God is always there alongside us wherever we go, whatever we are forced to confront in our lives. This will bring the healing presence of God to our midst, bringing healing to the body through the soul.

TWO

The Meaning of Illness and Healing in Jewish Tradition

udaism seeks to find meaning for our lives in every human encounter, for Judaism is more of a religion of this world than it is a religion of the next. And Jewish spirituality is a spirituality of the mundane as much as it is of the transcendent. Thus, it is not surprising to find that Jews look to illness as a spiritual teacher rather than relegating it exclusively to a challenge of the body that needs to be beaten and overcome. Judaism teaches that we should embrace illness as part of who we are because it is an integral part of the world in which we live. As a result, I believe that Judaism teaches us that one spiritually suffers through illness only when one cannot find meaning in it. This is an essential message that emerges from the Jewish path toward healing. It is also the lesson that is at the heart of the book of Job. It is not merely that Job underwent trauma and tragedy; rather, it is that Job suffers for no reason. Or worse, Job suffered because he became a pawn in the game played between God and evil. This is what has troubled people for centuries. His illness had no meaning, no redeeming value to it. That is why he suffered—and we along with him. When we can find meaning in our illness, suffering is overshadowed and we are in a better position to find spiritual healing at the same time.

As we discovered in the previous chapter, there are those who understand illness as punishment for one's sins. Others see illness simply as a mystery, one that, like God, is beyond human comprehension. Illness just seems to be a part of life's process, an inevitable part of living. We move between sickness and health throughout our lives. Writer Paul Cowan, who chronicled his struggle with leukemia in *The Village Voice* (1988), put it this way: "We are all going to enter the land of the sick at one time in our lives. The question is only when."

The world's population is not divided into people who are ill and people who are not. Rather, like most other aspects of our lives, we spend most of the time in the middle of the continuum and only deceive ourselves into believing that we are more fully on one side of the midpoint than the other. The goal of the healing process is to return to the center, rather than move fully over to one side, for that would not be in accord with human experience. Through the process of healing, one is brought back from the extremes and gains the feeling of being centered once again.

The Human Dimension

For me, the actual experience of illness is more important than is any theoretical construct in Judaism. The reality of illness undervalues any attempt to trace an understanding of illness in the history of Jewish thought; it's the human dimension that truly matters. However, I feel compelled to confront God as the source of suffering in a theoretical framework of a sound theological system. If I acknowledge God as the source of all life as I do, because of my faith, which has been bolstered by my direct experience with healing, I am more inclined to engage God as a healer rather than try to trace the root of anyone's illness necessarily to God. One seems almost irrelevant in the face of the other. The psalmist helps me here when teaching: "God forgives all your sins; God heals all your sicknesses" (Psalms 103:3). Thus, regardless of one's perspective on the cause of illness, the divine source for potential healing remains the same. Perhaps it does not really matter how classical Judaism or its pivotal thinkers look at illness. Instead, what is important is how Judaism considers the individual who is ill—and then helps him or her to galvanize resources to ameliorate the suffering.

The Bridge Between the Body and the Soul

When you are seriously ill, few things really matter. Issues that may have seemed so important only days or weeks before hold little value at all. The only topics that become relevant are those forces that will drive the patient toward healing, a foundation of family love, and a new-found respect for transcendent values. On the other hand, the simple pleasures of daily life and its small details take on enormous proportions, even those that may have seemed trivial in the past. Getting up each morning, though sometimes in itself a challenge, is an affirmation of the rabbinic teaching that we are reborn each day. Activities in our daily routines, categorized in the daily blessings of the morning worship service, now carry profound significance. Each breath we take, the liquids we drink, the food we eat: Each sip or mouthful is filled with blessing. This is especially true for things that we suddenly cannot do for ourselves. People and relationships take on a new level of meaning. Values that transcend time and place become central. While our focus may be on the body, at the same time the world of the spirit dwarfs the material world.

For the first time perhaps, the prayer *Asher yatzar,* which is traditionally said shortly after rising each morning and performing our normal routines of bodily function, provides us with incredible insight about our bodies and souls. In the prayer, we marvel at the mechanic functioning of our bodies, something we might previously have taken for granted. Most prayer books attempt to translate the core elements of the prayer rather creatively, using phrases like "intricate network of finely tuned organs and orifices" for *"nikavim nikavim chalulim chalulim."* I prefer the Hebrew to speak for itself—"holes, holes, tubes, tubes." It presents the reality of bodily function in the most basic way. When they are not functioning correctly, we feel clogged, bloated, indeed unable to stand before God. The *Asher yatzar* is followed by an acknowledgment of the unique nature of our souls in the *Elohai neshama.* This prayer affirms our belief in the purity of our souls and its source in God. While some may want to separate our bodies from our souls to make a distinction between our mortal bodies and our immortal spirits, this is not the Jewish way. We are our bodies in a measure equal to our souls. Our entire self is created in God's image: *b'tzelem Elohim.* As the liturgist eloquently stated, "The soul is yours and the body is your handiwork." These two prayers are joined together in the morning liturgy, connected by a short prayer directing us to study Torah, for it is in the study of Torah that we come to understand the relationship between body and soul. In the liturgy for *selichot,* the penitential prayers that precede Rosh Hashanah, we add this sentiment, "Have compassion on your handiwork."

Spirit is the bridge between mind and body that makes us human. As a result of our illness, we may not be able to stand upright to praise God—or to do anything else. Because of the heavy burden that a serious illness lays upon us, we may not even have the desire to stand upright, and we may resist praising God even when we are able to. However, the daily recitation of these prayers helps pave a path toward healing. It offers a prism through which to view our entire day and forces us to assume a posture that might otherwise be overlooked in our quest for healing—the alliance between the body and the soul. I find these moments in the morning when I stand alone with God to say my morning prayers to be among the most powerful of the day, much more significant than the afternoon or evening service, or even the proclamation of *Shema Yisrael* before lying down to go to sleep.

Jewish tradition understands feelings of resentment, as well. We are beckoned to take solace from what our ancestors taught us from their desert experience. The shards of the broken tablets were carried along with the unbroken ones in the ark of the covenant because God allows for a shattered world and for a people who are cracked, broken, and scared. But God also insists on going forward, continuing with what is broken and what is whole. Rabbi Rachel Sabath, a colleague of mine with whom I have taught spiritual texts, suggests that from this experience, we can learn to hold gently those broken parts of ourselves and others so that healing and renewed trust can be established, for it is trust that is broken when we are ill. When trust is shattered, not only is the relationship between the individual and God broken, but the hearts of the individuals involved are also shattered. How can one heal? Trust does not emerge on its own; it has to be built and rebuilt. As the psalms teach, "God is the healer of broken hearts."

Tamara Green, an active founding member of the National Center for Jewish Healing and someone who struggles with her body each day, offers her insight: "There must have been at Sinai some children of Israel who, like me, were physically broken and saw themselves as I did in those broken fragments of the covenant." She may not be able to find a way to mend her broken body—just as mystics understand that the shards of the broken world cannot be gathered together to recreate the world—but, she says, "I can gather up the scattered light." With that light, she can be healed. Even as our bodies are ill, we can acknowledge the transcendent nature of our souls, and the light to find our path in the world.

The Process of Illness

While there are those whose experience with illness might suggest the sentiment that "One day I was fine and the next day I was sick," illness almost always includes a downward spiral that extends over time. Jon, a good friend of mine, told me recently that he was feeling well when he suddenly found out that he had cancer. Upon reflection, he began to realize that he had not been feeling well over the previous few months. That's what drove him to the doctor for a "routine check-up." Just as one does not suddenly awaken old, generally one does not suddenly wake up sick. It is the physician's label of illness that typecasts us so abruptly. However, the physician's words are only a description of symptoms. They do not change who you were prior to the diagnosis. We often have taken neither our bodily cues nor the spiritual cues of our souls seriously. We ignore them, and at some point, the illness becomes impatient and takes control. Often it goes like this: A lack of spiritual light (or awareness) brings on sickness. This sickness presents itself physically in what might be described as, and often actually is, a blockage. In turn, this physical blockage causes spiritual blockage. It is this spiritual blockage that prevents the individual from receiving God's light.

To break this debilitating cycle and find healing, the healer—and often that healer is one's self—must find a way to free the entrapped spiritual powers in order to access God's divine light and its inherent healing. As a physician and rabbi, the Rambam, Moses Maimonides, understood this: "Physical health is a prerequisite for spiritual health, but a healthy body does not in itself produce a healthy spirit" (*Hilkhot Deot* 4:1). The Baal Shem Tov, founder of Hasidism, put it similarly, adding another element: "When a person is sick, his soul may also be weakened and therefore he cannot pray properly, despite the fact that he may be free of sin. Therefore a person must take care of his physical health" (Keter Shem Tov #231). The Torah agrees: "Take care of yourself and treat your soul diligently" (Deuteronomy 4:9).

Whenever I counsel people, I often ask them to retrace their lives during the weeks and months before the manifestation of their illness. As these stories unfold, I often detect a common theme. I can usually even identify some of the elements with them that presage this illness through a series of questions, and these become cues for getting them back on the path toward healing. When relationships are broken, they need to be repaired. When self-esteem is destroyed, it needs to be nurtured. Nevertheless, even when I have seen a theme repeatedly played out in what I describe as a downward spiritual spiral, the person often does not recognize it. I hear the echo of the prophet Ezekiel who cried out, "they have eyes that do not see and ears that do not hear" (Ezekiel 12:2). Just as they are not ready to listen to the hints their bodies and souls are offering them, they are likewise not ready to hear what I might have to say. I say it anyway, and have always taught my students to do the same. It is what I call an aggressive form of pastoral counseling. The normal protocol of "wait and see" will not suffice if I am to try to help prevent the onset of illness by addressing the themes that threaten to overwhelm a person. An outside observer might be moved to ask why so many bad things are happening to that person. The individual might even wonder such things to him- or herself, even if unable to articulate it. It is difficult to realize what is happening when you are in the middle of it. One thing leads to another. They are not random, dissociated episodes; they are connected in a chain of events. If we want to help someone find healing, we have to discover the interconnections that create the chain.

Just before my wife, Sheryl, was first diagnosed with cancer, our lives had developed a certain frenzied rhythm, a pattern of living that was hard to keep pace with. We worked hard. We played hard. We arose early in the morning and worked until late at night. We seldom just relaxed—we were busy paving a foundation for our future. While struggling with being devoted parents to our then young sons in addition to doing what was necessary to build successful careers, things always seemed to rush ahead of us, even as we attempted to reign them in and direct them. Sheryl's illness gave us the opportunity to reflect on what was happening so that we might learn from it and change what we were doing wrong. We had to stop everything so that she could find healing.

Sheryl clearly remembers racing through an airport one day, trying to catch a late night plane so she would not have to spend another night on the road. She recalls consciously struggling just to place one foot in front of the other. Exhausted from her work, she said that it was as if she were telling her legs what to do because they did not know how to work on their own. While she believed, as our teachers have suggested, that when we hold the words of Torah in our hearts they will carry us, the burden she carried was manifest in her overstuffed and overweight briefcase. On top of all this, her grandfather had recently died, and we had just gone through a scary episode that threatened the health of our younger son. We both learned that the rabbis were right when they wrote: "Three things take away a person's strength: fear, traveling, and sin" (Babylonian Talmud, *Gittin* 70a). We learned that these are not three separate items. Instead, one simply emerges in the guise of the other.

The Spiritual State of Sickness

The Hebrew word for sickness *(choleh)* is related to the word for emptiness or hollowness. That same word can also mean secular or profane. Thus, illness represents a state in which the lack of spirituality negatively impacts on the physical well-being of the individual. Sickness can ensue when the nonsacred side of one's life dominates and smothers the other side, potentially severing one's connection with God. The writer of Proverbs asks, "One's spirit strengthens oneself in one's illness, but who will lift up a broken spirit?" (Proverbs 18:4). The Malbim (Rabbi Meir Leibush ben Yechiel Michel) offers an answer: "It is the spirit that sustains the body. And even if there is sickness in the body, the spirit has great enough strength to support the illness, giving them strength to bear [the illness] and renew their courage. But if the spirit is broken [referring to spiritual sickness] who will lift it up? For then the sickness will affect the body too as it is written, 'A depressed spirit dries the bones'"(Proverbs 17:22). A psycho-spiritual commentary on the Biblical texts, Metzudat David, adds this explanation: "But when the spirit is broken by sadness and depression, who will lift it up? For the body does not lift it up to strengthen it; rather, it is the spirit that supports the body."

When people read in the Talmud, "The best of physicians are destined to go to hell" (*Kiddushin* 82a), they think this is an indictment against the medical profession. Rather, as the Maharsha (Rabbi Shmuel Eliezer ben Yehuda Levi of sixteenth-century Cracow) explains, it is a criticism against those doctors who think they are the "best of physicians" and rely only on themselves—rather than recognizing their partnership with the Divine and the spiritual side—as they do their healing work.

Remembering God

Each time I sit face-to-face with a person who is struggling with serious illness, a particular text from Exodus replays itself in my memory: "I am God your healer" (Exodus 15:26). I first studied it when I was a student rabbi and had to find the inner strength to make my first pastoral visits in the hospital. I was not sure that I had the inner spiritual reserve necessary, but this text became a *kavannah* for me, a sacred mantra that I repeated to myself each time I entered a hospital room, not knowing who or what to expect on the other side of the threshold. I continue to draw from it whenever I make such a visit.

In the midst of illness, it may be hard to remember how you felt before getting sick. Dr. Herbert Benson, a well-known leader in alternative or complementary medicine, suggests that the key to healing is to get the body and spirit to "remember (its) wellness," and he works with his patients to achieve this. Dr. Benson argues that if we can get ourselves to remember what it was like to feel healthy before becoming ill, we will then be able to move ourselves in the direction where healing takes place. At the same time, we have to block out everything that might prevent us from doing so. No negativity, no pessimism, only positive thinking. While this idea is still controversial in the medical community, it remains a leading idea in the area of alternative medicine. But what of the spiritual side of this "remembered wellness"?

Spirituality is focused on the relationship between God and an individual. Thus, the goal of spirituality is always to bring that relationship closer. Borrowing from the work of Rabbi Eugene Borowitz, North America's leading liberal Jewish theologian, it is called a *covenantal relationship,* one that mirrors the relationship established between God and the Jewish people at Sinai. In the midst of sickness, it might be difficult to remember the relationship one previously had with God, assuming that a relationship had been cultivated and nurtured at all. I believe that the key to remembering wellness, as per Dr. Benson, is to recall this original relationship with God. Here's how it works. I believe that all Jews possess "historical memory," the collective experience of the Jewish people that dates back to the covenant at Sinai. If so, regardless of whether or not they have ever accessed it, even if it has receded deep into the unconscious, then it may be possible to reach back into that memory and "remember" it. Pregnant women understand this idea rather well. Sarah, a neighbor of mine, told me that when she was pregnant, she kept misjudging how much room she would need to pass between two people or objects. She would constantly bump her belly into things, because she "remembered" her size before she was pregnant.

This is what the Passover seder attempts to accomplish in the family context. The Haggadah for the seder contains a step-by-step guide to help those sitting around the Passover table reach back and participate in the exodus again. It offers a model for the entire week of Passover and beyond. The Torah extends this idea: "If you listen to the voice of *Adonai* your God, and do what is right in God's eyes, and listen to God's mitzvot, and observe all of God's laws—all the diseases that I put upon Egypt, I shall not put upon you, for I, God, am your healer" (Exodus 15:26). For me, this "historical memory" is crucial to healing in Judaism. We bring the relationship with God back to the forefront of our consciousness by remembering it—and we bring healing along with it.

Drawing Closer to God

Rabbi David Wolpe, spiritual leader of Sinai Congregation in Los Angeles and the author of several bestsellers on spirituality and suffering, once wrote "Suddenly God seems closer to us when we are awake [sensitive to God's presence through our illness]." Regardless of our mental or physical state, we are all in need of healing. The Kotzker Rebbe, one of the most enigmatic of the Hasidic masters, taught that the only whole heart is one that has been broken; one cannot draw close to God unless one has been broken.

Rabbi Nachman of Breslov emphasized throughout his writings that all the spiritual pathways of healing are ultimately founded on faith. It is easy for the individual, especially at this time, to deny his or her faith, to argue that he or she is not a believer. But the process of healing is about developing and deepening one's faith wherever one begins. If you are not cured of the physical illness, it does not mean that you are not faithful enough or do not believe deeply enough. In the face of illness, our task is to search for God. Rabbi Nachman offers this advice: "When things are very bad, make yourself into nothing. Close your mouth and eyes—and you are like nothing. Sometimes you may feel overwhelmed by evil thoughts, finding it impossible to overcome them. You must then make yourself like nothing. You no longer exist, your eyes and mouth are closed. Every thought is banished. Your mind ceases to exist. You have nullified yourself completely before God" (Rabbi Nachman's Wisdom #279). According to this wisdom teacher, it is only through this process of abdicating of the ego *(bitul yesh)* that one can find healing.

Drawing closer to God involves four elements that are particularly important, especially for those who did not take the opportunity to foster such a relationship prior to illness. In the words of Dr. Eugene B. Borowitz: "God is a backdrop for healing, a backdrop for the processes by which people naturally induce the restoration of health." Illness focuses us on specific issues in a way like nothing else can because it exists in the shadow of death. It can be the means through which the individual is able to clear a path for the spiritual self. Admittedly, these four elements are difficult to establish when ill, but they are key to spiritual wholeness and thereby can lead to healing.

The first element is study. Divine light is reflected in the study of Torah; it illumines the dark corners of our souls and casts no shadows. "Torah is healing to all flesh" (Proverbs 4:22). Moreover, the rabbis have taught us that "The Holy Blessed One gave Torah to Israel. It is an elixir of life for the entire human body, as it is said, 'replenishment for your bones and healing to all flesh' (Proverbs 3:8)" (Babylonian Talmud, *Eruvin* 54a). The tradition attributes the writing of Proverbs to King Solomon and it is written, "It [Torah] is a tree of life for those who hold on to it" (Proverbs 3:18).

The second element is ritual. Ritual brings order into our lives, anchoring us as we travel through the tempest-tossed journey of life. It also offers us a vehicle to bring us closer to God and, in doing so, to self. According to Rabbi Nina Beth Cardin, author of *Tears of Sorrow, Seeds of Hope: A Jewish Spiritual Companion for Infertility and Pregnancy Loss* and a former member of the staff at the National Center for Jewish Healing, Judaism creates spiritual strength through the performance of mitzvot. They are the avenue through which we come into close contact with the Divine. Through the observance of rituals like Shabbat, divine light is brought from the spiritual realm into the physical realm. Shabbat comes weekly and its observance is considered equal to all other mitzvot. Out of Shabbat comes special ideas like Oneg Shabbat (joy of the Sabbath), for with joy comes healing.

Third is the element of prayer. Although I am not confident that I fully understand the power of prayer, I know that I have been captured by its force and experienced its potency. Prayer is not merely a function of sociology, that is, the act of Jewish folk coming together in community to articulate their aspirations. It is our way of communicating with God, of asking God to heal. The establishment of a regular prayer life helps to nurture the relationship with God. Rabbi Nachman of Breslov said, "Prayer is the main way in which to become connected to God. It is the gate through which we enter to God and come to know the Divine" (*Likutey Moharan* II, 84).

Last is the element that combines the others: Presence, of God and of others, in the form of community. The presence of persons and God is what the Jewish tradition describes as *bikur cholim,* visiting the sick. It is this visitation that makes an appreciable difference in the healing of a person. Some call this a social network. It sounds simple, rather obvious, but too many people are forced to endure their illnesses alone. These four elements are the crucial components to awakening the spirit and drawing close to God.

With this renewed sense of the spirit comes a dark side, what Rabbi Niles Goldstein, an ardent outdoorsman who sees Jewish spirituality most clearly in nature, calls "the dark side of spirituality." This includes fear of God, fear of the unknown, and, ultimately, fear of death. It is not the person who is afraid; it is something inside of him or her that must be identified and healed. Fear can be turned into awe and can bring us to a greater understanding of God. It can be a motivation to change our lives and move us toward repentance. The Baal Shem Tov taught, "The various fears a person has are really rooted in the hand of divine love and kindness that is stretched out to the individual. Such fears are sent out only to rouse one to fear God. When a person understands that fears are signs of God's kindness and are sent only to awaken him or her, fear turns into love—the love with which the individual can receive God's kindness—and as a consequence fear leaves the individual" (Keter Shem Tov I, #38).

The Will to Live

But there is much more to this thing called healing. I would like to suggest that it is the will to live that drives people forward, even in the face of life-threatening illness and disease. This form of unconventional healing has been manifest in our people's psyche throughout its history. While it is not exclusive to Jewish people, it is an exclusive characteristic of *the* Jewish people. This will to live is an indigenous ingredient of the people of Israel that is part of the collective memory we all carry. No matter what our people has encountered, it has fought to survive.

A few years ago, our region was struck by a terrible winter ice storm. Power lines fell throughout the state. Telephone lines were down. To the dismay of my children, even cable TV was out. We had a great deal of damage, including a willow tree in our backyard that had been split asunder. Even though the tree was hardy and had spread its roots over several years, it was no match for that winter assault—there was little left to it beyond its splintered trunk. While we cleaned up the debris, we decided to wait until spring before attempting to remove the trunk. To our wonderful surprise, with the first warm days of spring, the tree burst forth and sent new branches from every available space in its trunk. Today the tree, perhaps as a result of the brutal attack of the winter storm, magnificently covers a large part of our backyard and shields us from the summer sun. The Jewish people is similar to that tree. No matter how much it has been forced to endure, it has come back stronger than ever. This will to live courses through the blood of each of us and fuels us on our individual paths to healing. It explains the unexplainable and models the way for us.

From Illness toward Healing

Tamara Green believes scholars ask the wrong questions about healing when they focus on physical cure. She believes we should be asking, "Could I be spiritually healed even if I never got better physically? And if I was not to be cured, what did God expect of me?" Healing is more about helping the individual to achieve a peacefulness of spirit than it is about bodily cure. And it is this "peacefulness of spirit" that brings healing in its wake. This is possible even when bodily cure is not.

What Can We Learn from Illness?

As is usually the case, my wife's illness was devastating for our family. On reflection, however, because it drew us closer together—a necessary ingredient in fighting its ravages—we skipped over the personal midlife crises that affected many of our contemporaries. It may have been a horrible way to make the quantum jump, but we took it all the same. We had no choice.

Cynthia Parr experienced illness this way: "I learned that I had a brain tumor which was totally unrelated to the cancer. When I was first diagnosed with breast cancer, I took dozens of medical tests. One of them showed that I had a benign brain tumor the size of a man's fist pushing into my brain. I had absolutely no symptoms. After major brain surgery, the tumor was removed and I started my chemotherapy. I think about this every day. I actually thank God for the breast cancer that saved my life by revealing the brain tumor before it caused permanent damage or death."

Tamara Green learned something different: "One of the most painful lessons I have learned from this illness and the most difficult to come to terms with is not the possibility of dying from it, but the dailiness of living with it." She adds that suffering comes only when we do not learn. Rabbi Judah Hanasi observed: "Suffering is precious, so he took upon himself to suffer for thirteen years" (Babylonian Talmud, *Bava Metziah* 85a). Some do struggle with illness for a long time. For some, it is the time that they have felt closest to God. Job framed it this way: "Through my flesh, I see God" (Job 19:26).

The Torah records a middle-of-the-night struggle for Jacob. It is never clear who or what the patriarch was struggling with. Some say it was an internal struggle that was represented by the Torah as an angel. During the altercation, Jacob's thigh was injured and he developed a limp that he carried with him for the rest of his life as a reminder of his struggle. Toward morning, when the angel tried to leave, Jacob refused to let the angel go. Jacob relented only on the condition that the angel grant him a blessing. In the text, the price for this blessing seems to be the injury to Jacob's thigh. Like many of us who face life-threatening illnesses, Jacob was strengthened by his struggle with the angel—and he emerged with a blessing. Through an illness, though broken in body like Jacob, we can emerge whole through a blessing.

THREE

Healing Services:
An Introduction to Prayers for Healing

U pon opening this book, some readers will look first to this chapter, searching for a specific formula for immediate healing or an easily accessible how-to for healing prayers and services. They are less interested in the theoretical construct on which any of these prayers may be based. Readers want resources that promise to ease suffering and bring immediate healing either to themselves or to the one they love. Others—perhaps the strictly rational among us—may dismiss this chapter altogether or simply recognize the powerful poetry in its words. Many are colleagues who were trained to think, as I originally was, that things that did not make logical sense, what academics may call the metarational, was something we left behind as we progressed into the modern world. We were taught to distrust our senses and only to rely on rational thought as *the* measurement for truth. Later, we were taught only to look for a persuasive argument, data from research, and other indicators that prove prayers can bring healing. In a period of rebellious adolescence—it even carried me into adulthood—I bought into this approach, but I quickly left it behind on the narrow shoulders of the road called life. The rational has limits, but the spirit that goes beyond the rational is limitless. While this chapter does provide specific resources, it does provide a general approach to prayers for healing. But it begins with personal faith, the place at which I began when seeking prayers to bring healing to the body and to the spirit.

I believe in prayer and its power to heal. I also believe in the ability of prayer to heal the one who offers a prayer on another's behalf. Thus, prayer becomes circular, rather than one-directional. Nevertheless, for me, prayer is never about establishing a specific goal and getting there, even when the prayer is specifically for healing. Instead, prayer is about initiating a relationship with God and maintaining this relationship throughout one's journey in life, on the path toward healing and beyond. This relationship continually evolves, particularly in specific context and content. For the one who is engaged in routine prayer, the dialogue is maintained through three daily services, preferably in community, but in the privacy of self. According to Rabbi Abraham Joshua Heschel, one of the greatest theologians of the twentieth century, prayer is "a shift in the center of living—from self consciousness to self-surrender."[1] That surrender is to God. It includes a merging of self with the Divine into a sacred partnership, a covenant.

Physicians like Dr. Larry Dossey have attempted to gather together studies about the power of prayer to bring about cure. In his bestseller *Healing Words,* Dossey reviews numerous scientifically controlled studies in which prayer yielded significant change in the patient's well-being. At the very least, these studies open up windows into the world of the spirit.

During a transdenominational academic conference on

Jewish healing that I coordinated some years ago for three of the nation's major rabbinical seminaries, Dr. David Eisenberg of the Harvard Medical School made a presentation. He spent nearly an hour reviewing the lack of evidence to support any claim that prayer can lead to a cure. Perhaps willing to accept the possibility that prayer leads to spiritual healing but not physical cure, he picked apart arguments posed by best-selling authors such as Bernie Siegel, Andrew Weil, and his own teacher, Herbert Benson. While there seemed to be no hard evidence to support the hypothesis that prayer can lead to cure in the studies he analyzed, each offered a glimmer of light. There were too many changes that could not be explained, too many instances in which spontaneous healing occurred, but these were considered inconsistent, undependable, and impossible to duplicate in an experimental context. I was not persuaded, so I approached Dr. Eisenberg at the conclusion of his presentation. In a whisper, he confessed to me that he hated to offer presentations such as this one. When I probed him further, he responded, "Because in my heart, I still believe. I still believe." He prayed for the health of his son who had only a short time before been diagnosed with juvenile diabetes.

Shortly after my wife's first surgery, her surgeon discovered another suspicious lump in her neck during a follow-up examination. Instead of putting her through the time-consuming stress of additional diagnostic tests, he decided to schedule her for surgery once again. He determined that the suspected tumor would have to be removed regardless of the results of the test. About ten days later, during her scheduled surgery, the surgeon encountered difficulty finding the lump that he had previously documented. It had reduced in size from a walnut to a grain of rice. The doctor was surprised. My wife was not. She said, "I prayed. I visualized. I willed it to get smaller. And it did."

Prayers for healing take a multitude of forms. Some contain words, others conjure up visual images. Some are made from wordless melodies, and others are composed of silence. There are prayers that come from unexpected actions, such as dance. Such is the case in a story I heard that I later learned had been brought to light by Martin Buber. News was brought to Rabbi Moshe Leib that his friend, the rabbi of Berditchev, had fallen ill. During the Sabbath, Rabbi Leib said his friend's name over and over and prayed for his recovery. Then he put on new shoes made of morocco leather, laced them up tightly, and danced. A tzaddik who was present said, "Power flowed forth from his dancing. Every step was a powerful mystery. An unfamiliar light suffused the house and everyone watching saw the heavenly hosts joined in his dance."[2] Rabbi Wayne Dosick, in his book *Soul Judaism: Dancing with God into a New Era,* says that, "In our own confrontation with spiritual exile and physical illness, we have come to realize that a spontaneous, personal plea for healing—an unadorned, instinctive, involuntary supplication—is one of Judaism's oldest and most powerful soul-cries to God." Prayers for healing constitute a dance of the spirit, even when we do not move our feet!

"Please God, Heal Her, Please"

"El na, refa na lah" (Numbers 12:13). This is Moses' simple, heart-wrenching plea to God to heal his sister Miriam. It is the first example of a prayer for healing in our sacred literature and presents us with a paradigm to this day. With these five words, Moses gave over the care of his sister to the God whom he had followed from the day God called out to him from the midst of a burning bush, unconsumed by its own inferno. Moses did not let go of his responsibility toward Miriam. He continued to pray for her healing and well-being. According to one rabbi in the Talmud, Rabbi Eliezer, the short, sweet prayer of Moses on behalf of Miriam should be a model for all of our prayers of petition (Babylonian

Talmud, *Berakhot* 34a), not just those of healing. In times of real prayer, there is no need for verbosity or patronizing, no need for the multitude of fixed prayers that mark our tradition, although they have their rightful place and indeed have sustained our people through its many years of wandering. The utterance of our prayers, however framed, constitutes a statement of faith, a belief in our ability to call on God's power to heal.

It is important to note that Moses chose to utter his plea in the imperative. He used the command form of the verb (in Hebrew, *refa*—heal), an unusually strong choice for entreaty to God, softened only by a somewhat humble "please" (expressed as *na* in Hebrew). In this prayer, Moses stakes his claim in the context of his relationship with God, as if to say, "Heal her. Remember: It's part of the bargain we struck on Sinai, the covenant to which we both agreed. Our relationship is built on your ability to heal—and my willingness to believe." While some traditions use the form of gratitude as the model for faith, this covenantal form reflects the Jewish posture for faith. God and the individual are partners in the healing process. The individual does his or her part, and God is responsible to fulfill the divine part of the covenantal agreement.

Deuteronomy Rabbah, a midrash on this story of Miriam, explains it in a slightly different way. The author interprets Moses' plea *"El na,* please God" as if to say "God, you heal her. But if you do not, then I will heal her." The midrash describes it as more than a partnership. The rabbis believed, as we will explore in chapter 5, that we as individuals and as a community of individuals do possess the power to heal. However you choose to interpret this episode in the Torah, two things remain abundantly clear and are made manifest throughout Jewish history and replicated in our own experiences of living. First, God's presence in our lives brings healing. Second, any individual can impact the healing of another.

Use Moses' prayer for his sister Miriam as a model for your

own prayers of healing. Similarly, make them short and simple. Don't just rely on words that are formed by others, however poetic they may be. Simply speak from the heart. One of my favorite Hasidic stories involves a person who comes to the synagogue and recites only the Hebrew alphabet over and over again. The synagogue's caretaker is disturbed by this behavior and complains to the rabbi. In turn, the rabbi tells the caretaker: This is the most honest form of prayer heard in these sanctuary walls, because it comes from the heart. The individual is reciting the letters of the alphabet because that is all he knows, inviting God to weave the letters into the words of prayer.

Daily *Amidah* (*Rofeh Cholim*)

Each day, shortly after I arise, I say my morning prayers. It is part of my regular morning routine. Generally, it is still rather quiet in our house. Neither my spouse nor our children have yet awakened. I find it is just the right atmosphere to initiate my daily dialogue with the Divine. The emergence of a new day reconfirms my faith in God and provides me with the right context for such prayers. And three times each day, except on Shabbat and holidays, I include in my prayers—specifically in the *Amidah,* in the section called *Rofeh Cholim,* the healer of the sick—the names of those for whom I ask for God's healing. Some days the list is quite long and as I say each name aloud, I make a mental image of the person. I review his or her relationship with me, the times that we have shared. I want to make sure that God takes the time to listen, as I take the time to offer the prayer. While there are days in which my concentration for prayer (what the tradition calls *kavannah*) may be elusive, I force myself to shut out all thoughts that distract me when I am ready to pray for the health of another, and I properly direct my spiritual energies heavenward.

Since the personal prayers of petition are part of the central prayer in all Jewish worship services—the *Amidah,* also known as *ha Tefillah* or the *Shemoneh Esreh*—we are obligated to offer prayers of healing nearly every time we pray. And as we pray, we hold the names of those for whom we seek God's healing in our hearts and in our minds. We also ask for guidance and insight for those entrusted with their care. Such efforts at community healing often do work. In his inspirational book *God Was Not in the Fire,* Rabbi Daniel Gordis says that the prayer book reminds us of the small, significant moments of redemption in our lives, establishing a belief system that acknowledges that we can find the courage and strength to continue on the spiritual quest that is so central to Jewish life. The *Amidah* expresses the conviction that we will find such courage as we move toward greater dreams and hopes. Rabbi Gordis reminds us that the *Amidah* wants us to reexperience those moments of healing and of hope, and to gain the courage to continue our struggle for growth and insight from those memories. That is why in the *Amidah* the prayer for redemption is followed by two concrete examples of ways in which we have been redeemed.

Healing prayers are part of an ongoing dialogue with the Divine. They are not reserved just for special times or synagogue moments, although I do include them at those times as well. Perhaps it is arrogance of a sort to suggest that God would listen to our individual prayers, but I offer them nonetheless. I also make sure to join them to the collective prayers of my community whenever I am able to do so, and I urge others to do the same.

Below you will find the standard prayer for healing included in the daily *Amidah.* You may find some variation in translation from prayer book to prayer book, but the major thrust of the prayer remains the same: God has a reputation as a healer. We have all experienced healing in the past in our personal lives, even from minor illnesses when our bodies did not function properly.

Similarly, our people has experienced healing in the form of redemption. Therefore, the one who offers the prayer asks God to
act according to the divine reputation, what is often referred to as
God's name, and heal a specific person or persons whom we remember by name.

> Heal us, *Adonai*, and we shall be healed. Help us and save
> us for You are our song. Grant perfect healing for all our
> afflictions.

> On behalf of someone ill, you may add:

> May it be Your will, *Adonai* our God and God of our an-
> cestors, to send perfect healing, of body and of soul, to
> _____ along with all others who are stricken.
>   For You are the faithful and merciful God of healing.
> Praised are You, *Adonai*, healer of the people Israel.

What to Expect
from Healing Services

The prayer book might be considered a history book of the
Jewish soul. While there is a specific liturgy for nearly all of Jewish
life and there are specific prayers for healing that are inserted in
various contexts, there is no fixed, independent liturgy for healing
services. Perhaps it is just too new of a phenomenon. However,
since the motivation and desire to seek healing from God is not
new, it seems more likely that Jewish liturgists have stayed away
from fixing a liturgy for healing. They recognized people's desire
to allow their prayers to flow directly from their hearts without
any of the restrictions that a prepared liturgy places on them.
Thus, it gives those who are interested in developing a *matbeah
tefillah* (a structure or rhythm for prayer) a great deal of freedom

and flexibility to develop a liturgy without measuring it against any standard.

Those of us who are used to a fixed liturgy—and find comfort in it—may find this surprising and even uncomfortable. Classic Judaism rejected a fixed liturgy for healing in order to offer the worshiper some flexibility in worship between fixed and spontaneous prayer. Even the *Amidah,* discussed above, was really only intended to provide themes as guidelines for worship, but the selected prayers of individual rabbis were recorded and repeated over time until they became commonplace and eventually fixed, often at the expense of personal prayers. A healing service can provide the individual with a structured time and place for focused prayer that draws on a mixture of traditional Jewish liturgy and nontraditional texts and activity. This mixture reflects the service that connects us to classic Jewish tradition and modern modes of worship.

As was expressed in chapter 1, the service of healing is more reflective of the theology of the worshiper than of the worship itself. Some worshipers will come to a service (or pray individually) expecting that God can fulfill all prayers; others will seek God as a source of comfort. Still others may see God as part of the great life force of creation that can aid healing. There will be those who will find comfort and healing in the gathering of a group rather than its focus on the Almighty. We can gain strength in facing adversity with the support of others. Few of us come to healing services for any one of these reasons alone. Instead, they all serve the purpose of bringing us to the path toward healing. As Rabbi Nancy Flam suggests, "Almost all services have one thing in common: the desire to create out of a gathering of discrete individuals in pain a community of comfort."[3]

Healing services belong to the people who prepare them and participate in them. They are not fodder for criticism or critique. When you participate in a healing service, whether on an individual or community basis, leave your analytic mind and any penchant for cynicism outside the sanctuary. Most healing services include a variety of elements that are discussed below. Use this outline as the starting point and then let your soul soar. As the rabbis have been known to say, "Words that come from the heart enter the heart."

Proposed Service of Healing Outline

While in most contexts, rabbis and cantors make decisions regarding worship services and the choices of liturgy, the service for healing is often arranged by lay participants. The material below is included for your information, should you have the desire or inclination to do so. This suggested outline is intended to familiarize you with the concept of a specific healing service; even if you don't attend one on a communal basis, it will provide a guideline for individual prayers.

1. A ritual of transition, such as handwashing, often introduced and/or accompanied by a *niggun*
2. The connection of Body and Soul (*Asher yatzar* and *Elohai neshama*)
3. Expressing gratitude and thanksgiving for the miracles of daily living
4. A *vort*, a word of Torah
5. Prayers for Healing: *Mi Sheberakh*
6. Reflections and Personal Prayers
7. Closing Prayers, the Priestly Benediction

1. A Ritual of Transition

Healing services should begin gently. Service leaders often introduce the service with a wordless chant (a *niggun,* made famous by Hasidism). In addition, some people like to include a

specific ritual and experiment with the washing of hands, often performed by another person, as was the case with the ancient priests.
Immersion in water marks various points of ritual transformation,
such as when a woman enters the ritual bath following menstrua-
tion or as part of the process for conversion to Judaism for both
men and women. This ritual takes its cue from Isaiah 12:3: "You
shall draw forth water with joy from the wells of salvation."

2. The Connection of Body and Soul
(Asher Yatzar and Elohai Neshama)

Asher Yatzar

In the morning, after we rise, we offer a prayer that affirms our
ongoing relationship with our creator and expresses gratitude for
our bodies' ability to function properly. This prayer is coupled
with Elohai neshama, a similar prayer that recognizes God as the
source of life who renews our souls each day. Rabbi Neil Gillman,
Professor of Jewish Philosophy at the Jewish Theological
Seminary of America and author of The Death of Death:
Resurrection and Immortality in Jewish Thought, has taught in refer-
ence to this prayer, "The normal functioning of our body is as
miraculous as the angel's ascent into the flames of the sacrifice [in
the story of Samson, Judges 13:21]. We commonly ignore that association because we take our bodily functions for granted—
until, of course, our bodies cease to function as we expected and
we are shocked into awareness of just how wondrously God has
fashioned them."[4]

This is a standard text that describes the unique system of
our bodies:

> Praised are You, Adonai our God, Creator of the universe,
> who has made the human form in wisdom and created in it
> a system of openings, arteries, glands, and organs that is

marvelous in structure and intricate in design. Should only one of them fail to function by being blocked or open, it would be difficult to stand before You. Wondrous fashioner and sustainer of life, source of our health and our strength, we give You thanks and praise.

Elohai Neshama

Like its companion prayer *Asher yatzar,* the *Elohai neshama* acknowledges the existence of the soul and God as its creator. The text intentionally makes use of the same verbs, in the same order, as found in the Torah in the story of creation in Genesis. Some say that *Asher yatzar* and *Elohai neshama* are actually two parts of the same prayer. *Elohai neshama* is part of the standard morning liturgy. Implicit in the prayer is the belief that each night one goes to sleep and God takes back the soul, returning it in the morning, renewed and refreshed. According to the rabbis, sleep imitates death. Thus, the prayer suggests that the soul separates at death and is reunited at the end of days. According to a midrash, God assigns four guardian angels to look after us while we are sleeping and while God is renewing our souls. Yet, when we go to sleep each night, we know not whether we will arise in the morning. This prayer gratefully acknowledges this process of renewal, for when the soul is returned to us, unlike when we lend, say, a lawn mower to a neighbor, it comes back undamaged. Much to our delight and surprise, the soul is returned to us in better shape than it was the prior night.

My God, the soul which you have placed within me is pure. You have created it. You have formed it. You have breathed it into me. You preserve it within me and You will one day take it from me and restore it to me in time to come. So long as my soul is within me, I make acknowledgment before you, my God and God of all generations. Praised are You, God, who restores my soul each day, that I may once again awaken.

3. Expressing Gratitude and Thanksgiving for the Miracles of Daily Living

As part of our morning prayers we recite a series of daily blessings. Below is the standard list, adapted somewhat (as they have been by the Reform, Reconstructionist, and Conservative movements) to reflect greater gender sensitivity. Each blessing begins with the standard form for blessing (*Barukh ata Adonai . . .*), which for me indicates the initiation and affirmation of a dialogue with the Divine. However, in the context of a creative healing service, we should feel free to explore alternative formats for initiating this dialogue. Some may choose to introduce these blessings with an alternative formula, such as the one proposed by Marcia Falk (Let us bless the source of life, creator of all . . .) or with those found in Jewish renewal circles (We praise the one, source of eternity . . .). The former emphasizes human action. The latter uses feminine language to describe the manifest attributes of the Holy One.

> Praised is the source of life, who has made me in the Divine image.
> Praised is the source of life, who has led me to my Jewish heritage.
> Praised is the source of life, who has made me free.
> Praised is the source of life, who opens the eyes of those who would not see.
> Praised is the source of life, who establishes firm ground amidst the waters.
> Praised is the source of life, who provides for all my needs.
> Praised is the source of life, who girds us with courage.
> Praised is the source of life, who brings freedom to the captive.
> Praised is the source of life, whose power lifts up the fallen.
> Praised is the source of life, who makes firm each person's steps.
> Praised is the source of life, who gives strength to the weary.

4. A Vort, *a Word of Torah*

The rabbis teach that the presence of God can be found wherever there are those who study Torah. Furthermore, the study of sacred texts is a form of prayer as it acknowledges the ultimate source of these texts. I believe that the Torah does not exist unless and until we are prepared to engage the text. It is within our power to provide the voices for Torah to be renewed in our midst. The Torah is not merely the scroll that is housed in the ark; rather, it is the ongoing revelation of God to the Jewish people, which is admittedly sometimes difficult to hear because of all the noise in the world (and sometimes we have to admit that we are the cause of this "interference"). Moreover, Torah represents the spiritual life story of the Jewish people as its relationship with God evolved over time and continues to do so. I believe that healing is part of the struggle to find the path to God and get closer to the Divine.

Some choose to begin their encounter with sacred texts with the traditional blessing contained in the morning liturgy for the study of Torah—Praised are You, *Adonai* our God, sovereign of the universe, who makes us holy with mitzvot and instructs us to busy ourselves in the words and works of Torah. While we can teach our own Torah, there are many examples in the ancient Torah that can teach us about healing and are worthy of exploration. For example, the prophet Elijah was known as a personal healer. The Bible tells us that he increased the food supply of Zarepthath's widow so that she and her young son would not starve to death during a drought (1 Kings 17:11). And when the child fell ill with "no breath left in him," Elijah called out to God that the child might be healed: "*Adonai,* my God, let this child's life return to his body." By calling on the power of God, the child was revived and lived (1 Kings 17:17, 21ff).

Elijah's disciple Elisha demonstrated healing powers as well. He provided food for people where there was none (2 Kings

4:38–44) and continually filled the empty jugs of a widow so that she could repay her debts (2 Kings 41:1–7). And like his teacher, he healed the son of a Shunamite woman (2 Kings 4:32–37).

5. *Prayers for Healing:* Mi Sheberakh

As a child, I would often hear my grandparents talking with their peers about one among them who was ill. The comment from my grandfather was always, "I will make them a *Mi Sheberakh,*" referring to a specific prayer for healing. While we usually say these prayers on behalf of those who are ill, there are many contexts in which a *Mi Sheberakh*—referring to the first Hebrew words of the prayer "The one who blesses"—may be offered. Nevertheless, the importance of this context has given rise to referring to the healing version of this prayer as <u>the</u> *Mi Sheberakh*. It is indeed the central Jewish prayer said for those who are ill or recovering from illness or accidents. Expressing a holistic view of human nature, the prayer asks for a complete healing *(refuah shleima)*. With it we pray for physical cure *(refuah haguf)* as well as spiritual healing *(refuah hanefesh)*. We ask for blessing, compassion, restoration, and strength within the community of others facing illness as well as for all Jews, and for all human beings.

Traditionally, the *Mi Sheberakh* is said in the synagogue when the Torah is read because Jewish tradition requires a *minyan* (prayer quorum). The *Mi Sheberakh* is usually chanted by the cantor. In some congregations, the names of the ill are mentioned individually. However, in many synagogues it is the practice to invite people forward so that the names of those who are ill can be spoken aloud and one *Mi Sheberakh* is chanted. Many communities are experimenting with different models.

With the *Mi Sheberakh* we do not pray for people based on their own merits. We pray for them in connection with the accounts of our righteous ancestors, Abraham, Isaac, and Jacob (note: we add Moses, Aaron, David, and Solomon for a sick person). We may include our foremothers Sarah, Rebecca, Leah, and Rachel or Ruth, Yael, Esther, and Miriam. If the patient cannot be at services in person, a close relative or friend might be called to the Torah for an honor, and the one leading services will offer this prayer, filling in the name of the one who is ill along with the names of his or her parents. (Traditionally, the person uses the name of the mother rather than the father, as is customary in most other Jewish ritual contexts and particularly in Torah honors.)

Mi Sheberakh
Music by Debbie Friedman
Lyrics by Debbie Friedman and Drorah Setel
(based on the traditional Jewish prayer for healing)
Mi sheberakh avotenyu
Mekor habrakha limoteynu
May the source of strength
Who blessed the ones before us
Help us find the courage
To make our lives a blessing.
And let us say: Amen.
Mi sheberakh imoteynu
Mekor habrakha lavotenyu
Bless those in need of healing
With refuah shleima:
The renewal of body,
The renewal of spirit.
And let us say: Amen.

6. Reflections and Personal Prayers

At this time in the service, some may want to share their personal stories of illness and healing, or of those for whom they offer care. It is also a time for the private to merge with the public, the constant *tzimtzum* (expansion and contraction) common to Jewish prayer services where there is a place for private and personal prayers in addition to communal worship. Some may want to take this opportunity to vocalize a personal prayer or reflect on a personal struggle.

7. Closing Prayers, the Priestly Benediction

At the end of a communal service, the goal is to bring about closure and hope. In some services, the prayer leader offers the priestly benediction or calls on an inspirational text from Jewish sacred literature. Others invite participants to offer a blessing for one another, using the framework of the priestly benediction, but adding their own words of blessing.

> May God bless you and keep you.
> May the light of God's presence shine on you and be gracious to you.
> May God's presence be near to you and bless you with peace.

FOUR

Psalms of the Heart

Psalms form the heart of Jewish prayer, so we find either entire psalms or selected texts throughout Jewish liturgy. In addition, they are recited in various contexts in Jewish life, particularly when someone is ill. It is not unusual to find someone sitting at the bedside of a friend or loved one who is sick, reciting psalms as a means of maintaining the dialogue with the Divine. They are a crucial part of my personal prayer life. I linger on them as I make my way through the daily liturgy, and they often eclipse my more formal prayers as I meditate on individual verses or words.

Reflecting both our pain and our longing, the psalms affirm this posture: "God will sustain him [and we add: her] in the sickbed" (Psalm 41:4). There are those who sit alone and recite psalms. Many people keep the Book of Psalms by their bedside to read prior to going to sleep.

The words of the psalms grew out of the experience of people. They were not necessarily written by the great liturgical poets of the ages, as scholars would have us believe. I think they were written by people just like us who were struggling with everyday life, people who found the words to express what others felt. Some rabbis have suggested that they provide the one who is ill with a voice when he or she might otherwise be silent. Psalms give us permission to say things we are either unwilling or unable to say. The last psalm, Psalm 150, takes this notion one step further as it invites us to praise God with instruments, to praise God with the very gift that God gave us to keep us alive—our breath. So when words do not work, when there is nothing left to be said, when you are entirely spent and unable to speak any further, let your breath alone speak for your heart. Psalms also have a unique way of calming the spirit, a necessary step on the path toward healing. But illness is also a time for original prayers and poetry of healing. Let the psalmist only initiate the speaking.

How to Use the Psalms

While Psalms may be considered the "chap book" of the entire Jewish people, some people consider the psalmist (whom the tradition names as David) to be the poet laureate of the Jewish people. Others, like me, believe that the psalms were written by individuals much like ourselves who cry out in their pain to God, asking for support and healing. While they may contain profound and complex religious issues, they are not the stuff of the ivory tower. They are the real feelings of the people.

I avoid explicit analysis and strict interpretation of the psalms and psalm-texts mentioned below. The beauty and majesty of the psalms are manifest in their equivocality, not in the specific understanding of individual verses or even entire psalms. In some cases, it is the rhythm of the language alone that offers us internal calm. Below are my suggestions for how the psalms can be used to effect healing and provide comfort and inspiration, as I have gleaned from my personal practice and from the depths of Jewish tradition. The psalms referred to in this chapter are just a beginning. Feel free to take out the entire Book of Psalms (available either as a separate volume or in any *Tanakh,* Jewish Bible), and read them.

1. Read the psalms slowly and deliberately. This is different reading than what you might be used to. Savor each word. Pause between verses and whole psalms. Read them in the morning when you awaken to help frame your day, and before you sleep to help you find your way through the night. Read them at the bedside of the one who is ill.

2. Choose one specific line as your *kavannah* for the day. Repeat it over and over until it becomes part of you. As you prepare to do something, whether mundane or sublime, speak the line aloud. If there is a known melody that accompanies it, let the notes guide you. If not, sing out the melody that is inscribed on your soul.

3. Choose a psalm and repeat it aloud or say it in the presence of (or in the name of) the one who is ill. Continue to repeat the psalm until one line flows into the next, until the end of the psalm becomes its beginning.

4. Write out the words of one of Rabbi Nachman's psalms (see below), the one that speaks most to you, and place this next to your bed or the bed of the one who is ill. Invite visitors to speak the words of the psalm aloud.

5. Choose a psalm that reflects how you feel or what you desire and then write out the same sentiments in your own words so that your words might become a sacred text.

Rabbi Nachman's Psalms

Rabbi Nachman of Breslov believed that inherent in the psalms is what he called a "comprehensive remedy" or general healing, a *tikkun klali.* As a result, he selected a series of psalms that he believed brought healing. This series included Psalms 16, 32, 41, 42, 59, 77,

90, 105, 137, and 150. As Rabbi Nachman wrote in the introduction to his collection:

> The way of the comprehensive remedy is to first work to uplift and enhance the mind and intellect so as to draw cleansing from there to rectify all of one's failures. This comprehensive remedy must be effected first and then all of the individual details will be remedied by themselves. It may be that the comprehensive remedy is higher and more exalted than the individual remedy for each detail. Nevertheless, the remedy for each one depends on bringing down cleansing from the soul and spirit. The mind can only be elevated through the comprehensive remedy. This is why it is first necessary to go the higher level, the level of the comprehensive remedy, so as to rectify and elevate the mind. Then everything else will also be remedied as a matter of course. (*Likutey Moharan* 1:29, 1–2)

Psalm 16
This psalm is written from the perspective of one who is ill and suffers, who is in need of God's constant reassurance and support. It is a psalm of hope, one that is built around the core of *shiviti* (I keep God continually before me). It concludes with a request for God's direction for our lives.

Psalm 32
This psalm anticipates the time when the person who recites it has recovered from illness. By putting you in an anticipatory frame of mind, it helps you move in that desired direction.

Psalm 41
This psalm is a meditation on suffering. By confronting personal pain and anguish, the psalmist struggles through it. In doing so, the psalmist provides a model for us to emulate.

Psalm 42
This psalm is an outpouring of the soul's anguish, whose only reconciliation can be found in one's personal faith in

God. Its conclusion provides us with perspective as we engage in an ongoing encounter with our illness: "Though my bones feel crushed and my soul is disquieted, I will yet praise God, my ever present hope."

Psalm 59

In this psalm, the writer is able to face tragedy and despair, and through personal faith, transform that experience into a song of gratitude and thanksgiving. The psalmist suggests that we do the same.

Psalm 77

The psalmist is able to gain strength by remembering the past deeds of God and the relationship of the Divine with our ancestors. Just as God took our people through the desert, God will also accompany us on our journey through the wilderness of illness.

Psalm 90

In this psalm, the writer reflects on the challenges of everyday living. This is especially important as we attempt to establish a semblance of a normal routine following our encounter with the angel of death.

Psalm 105

Offering two paths to healing, it advises us to take control of our illness by praising God.

Psalm 137

This psalm expresses our pain, our yearning to return to a "Jerusalem state-of-mind," as well as a physical state of being. Because of the deep pain it expresses, it is said annually on Tisha B'av.

Psalm 150

This psalm is included in the daily service and brings closure to its "verses of song." Since words are inadequate to express what we feel, we turn to instruments. The last verse sums it up: "When there is nothing left to say, no more music to play, let our spirits be our instruments of praise. Let our very breath, the breath that was given to us by God, be used to praise God."

Inspirational Psalms and Kavannot

The Twenty-third Psalm is undoubtedly the most well-known of the psalms, even among Jews who do not frequent the synagogue. It finds its way into many life experiences. The simply beauty of its words (in both Hebrew and English) and sentiments reflects its majesty. Another lesser-known psalm that inspires hope is Psalm 121, which reflects our faith in God as our source of abiding strength. As a result, its words are repeated (often sung) throughout our lives. I often sing it to myself as I walk through the streets or anticipate a rough day ahead.

Kavannot are bits of sacred texts that are used to help individuals find their center. They are often used to help people focus, particularly as they prepare for prayer, rituals, and life cycle events. I use them frequently, primarily in Hebrew, to help me move from the routine into the extraordinary. While *kavannot* can come from a variety of sacred sources, the ones suggested below are taken exclusively from the Book of Psalms. I sing them to myself in the early morning as I prepare for prayer, on the way to work, and even after I have washed my hands prior to reciting my blessing over bread. These texts promote healing and are particularly helpful during recovery from surgery, during hours of diagnosis and laboratory tests, and during chemotherapy.

> I do not fear the thousands of people
> that have set upon me, all around.
> Rise up, *Adonai!* Save me, my God!
>
> *Psalm 3:7–8*

> Do not chastise me while you are angry, *Adonai,*
> do not chastise me while You are furious (with me).
> Have mercy on me, for I am weak.
> Heal me, *Adonai,* for my very bones tremble,
> My entire being shakes terribly,

while you, *Adonai*—how long?
Turn to me *Adonai;* save my life.

Psalm 6:2–5a

The Torah of *Adonai* is pure, reviving the soul.

Psalm 19:8

One thing I ask of *Adonai*,
One thing I seek:
To dwell in the house of *Adonai*
All my days,
To behold *Adonai*'s pleasantness
and to be reflective in God's sanctuary.

Psalm 27:4

Have hope in *Adonai*
Be strong and your heart will be strengthened.
Have faith in *Adonai*.

Psalm 27:14

To you, *Adonai*, I call
and to *Adonai* I appeal:
Hear, God, and have compassion on me,
God—be my help.

Psalm 30: 9, 11

Create for me a pure heart, God;
And renew within me the right spirit.
Don't cast me away from Your presence,
Don't take Your holy spirit away from me.

Psalm 51:12–13

O my strength, to You I sing hymns;
for God is my haven, my faithful God.

Psalm 59:18

Hear my prayer to You, *Adonai,*
be at a favorable time;
God, in Your loving abundance of kindness,
Answer me, with the truth of Your deliverance.

Psalm 69:14

Whenever I have said, "My foot has slipped,"
Your loving abundance of kindness, *Adonai,* has
    supported me.

Psalm 94:18

Adonai, hear my prayer.
Let my cry come before You.
Do not hide Your face from me
in my time of trouble;
turn Your ear to me;
when I cry, answer me quickly.

Psalm 102:2–3

In distress, I've called out to God,
God answered me by setting me free.

Psalm 118:5

FIVE

✡

The Role of the Individual and the Community

The Power of the Individual

Out of a profound respect for the potency of the individual in Jewish tradition, Judaism imposes an obligation on every person to visit the sick. Additionally, Jewish law mandates that this is one of the few obligations that may be "performed without measure" (*Mishnah Peah* 1:1). Unlike most mitzvot whose limits should not be exceeded, this mitzvah should be continuously performed without regard to frequency or duration. It is so important that it is included as part of the study material in the morning worship service as a reminder of what we are obligated to do during the day ahead.

Each individual is part of the healing equation. But healing is not a consolidated process nor is the power to heal in the hands of any single person. Individuals visit the sick, but their visits are best viewed as part of a personal responsibility in the context of a community response. Such visits help to address the reality of isolation and alienation felt by someone who is ill.

Thus, healing involves the persistent actions of a variety of people, all focused on the well-being of the one who is sick. Think about your illness or that of the one you love. Consider how the very presence of a visitor changes the atmosphere. As a rabbi, I realize, during my frequent visits, that by bringing the frenzy of the outside world with me, just my presence reminds people of the world that they are indeed still a part of—and can return to.

The rabbis of the Talmud promoted the notion of how a visit can relieve suffering. Rabbi Abba ben R. Chananiah taught that the visit to an individual who is ill takes away one-sixtieth of the person's suffering (Babylonian Talmud, *Nedarim* 39b). If that is the case, reasoned his critics, then a visit by 60 people would alleviate all of the suffering. Rabbi Chananiah explains that each visit removes one-sixtieth of the suffering that remains from the previous visitor (starting with the first). As individuals, we may be unable to fully alleviate suffering, but we can do a great deal to minimize it. The first visit may be the most healing (if we measure in quantities), but each visitor contributes.

Elsewhere in the Talmud, Rav Huna asserts that enough love might entirely eradicate the pain (*Nedarim* 30a). This is a powerful theory. How much love would it take to eradicate the pain of suffering, and are we capable of giving that much? Are we able to abdicate the self so fully that we can give of our entire being? In any case, just as we have learned that growing from the experience of illness can alleviate suffering, here we come to understand that the expression of love by others can similarly alleviate pain.

Rabbi Akiva had an alternative approach. Once, after visiting one of his student followers who had become ill, he cleaned and straightened up the student's room. The young man then revived. According to the report in the Talmud, this simple act of care and dignity cured the patient of his ills (*Nedarim* 40a). But Rabbi Akiva also wanted to teach his colleagues, who refused to lower themselves to visit a mere student, that differences in social status between the visitor and patient are irrelevant. He went so far as to say that one who does not visit the sick sheds his (or her) blood. These Talmudic anecdotes demonstrate the healing power of relationships in the context of visiting the sick—an obligation that is acted on by individuals and generally affirmed by others in the community.

Rabbi Yochanan ben Zakkai was well-known among his peers for his power to heal. One day, ben Zakkai himself fell ill. Just as he had been taught, colleague Rabbi Hanina visited him. After speaking to the stricken sage, Hanina held out his hand and ben Zakkai stood up. Following this episode, Hanina's students asked, "If Yochanan ben Zakkai was such a great healer, why couldn't he heal himself?" The rabbis answered with a metaphor, "Because the prisoner cannot free himself from prison" (*Berakhot* 5b).

When we visit those who are ill, we actually share the burden of their illness, much like the priest did with those who were stricken in the Torah with *tza'arat,* the mysterious disease that struck both the body and the soul. In the Torah, the priest was only able to heal the stricken Israelite when he took on the *tza'arat* himself. Similarly, we can only bring healing to others when we are prepared to share the emotional, spiritual, and physical burdens. It is what the rabbis of the Talmud really meant when they taught about "lifting" one-sixtieth of the burden.

Generally, we tend to think only of the one who is ill as being in need of a therapeutic visit. Our attention is focused on the patient. However, the caregiver also needs such a visit, for he or she often takes on responsibilities of daily life that might have previously been shared. During Sheryl's illness, there were those who understood that obligation as well, making sure that I looked after myself and helping me with the children, even as I tried to maintain the normalcy of our home.

Moving from
Individual to Community

The minimal requirement for a community is defined by Jewish tradition as a *minyan,* a prayer quorum of ten. It provides a structure for Jews to get together, to nurture and support one another in times of need and celebration. This requirement, with origins in the Torah, shows that in their wisdom, the rabbis understood the power of the community in bringing forth healing. The number of people assembled to form a community even limits which prayers can be recited in a prayer service in the traditional Jewish community, the context for communal prayers for healing. Thus, the assembling of people as a community has a profound impact on healing.

Jonathan, a friend of my sons Jesse and Avi, tells me that he feels honored whenever he is asked to complete a *minyan.* It means that his presence is important to help heal someone who is ill, especially when he may feel otherwise helpless in doing so. But he is far from helpless. Because we have a personal stake in the healing process, we have a personal responsibility to "make *minyan,*" rather than waiting until we are called.

Visiting the Sick

Bikur cholim (visiting the sick) is part of the healing "delivery system" of the individual and the community. It is an indispensable element in the healing formula. Rabbi Nancy Flam and her former colleagues at the National Center for Jewish Healing suggest that we visit the sick for a variety of reasons: to provide comfort; to offer a compassionate presence; to bring a sense of Jewish community by acting as its representative; to help the person see him- or herself as whole and complete (by being seen that way by the visitor); to help the person to express him- or herself authentically; to offer distraction from the worries and troubles of illness; and finally, to communicate to the person that he or she is remembered and missed by their former context.

We visit others in fulfillment of the divine directive to love our neighbors as ourselves. This is the primary motivation for much of what we do when it involves our relationships with other people. So it comes as no surprise that the incentive for visiting the sick originates from the same source. We should love others because they are like us, not only because we ourselves may fall ill and would want others to come visit us. It is part of the shared vulnerability of the human condition. It reminds us of our own mortality, our own finitude. We are obligated to value the other (particularly if illness causes a change in the role of the sick individual) as we value ourselves.

This notion of a shared vulnerability is expressed in this well-known Hasidic story. A rebbe approached a factory owner in the midst of a frigid Russian winter to solicit funds for charity. Despite the severe cold, the rebbe insisted that the factory owner come to the outside gate to meet him. As they discussed the rebbe's requests, the owner became more and more uncomfortable. Finally, he violated his own rules of respect for this great rabbi by demanding that they go inside where it was warm to discuss the matter further. The rebbe hastened to explain why he had insisted on meeting outside in the cold. "The poor suffer greatly in the winter because they lack warm clothing and firewood. If we met inside, you would, of course, be generous. If we stand outside, however, you will feel the cold and, understanding the pain of the poor, will be even more generous."

When to Visit

Traditional Jewish authorities have developed a series a guidelines to help guide those who want to visit someone who is ill. While modern sensibilities may not allow everyone to immediately

warm to some of these ideas, we can relate to the sentiments expressed by the rabbis, which are worthy of exploration so that they
can be adapted to one's own level of comfort.

According to Jewish tradition, relatives and friends who are ac-
customed to visiting someone should do so as soon as the person
hears that the person is ill. Strangers, however, should wait until the
third day of the illness. While members of the community are obligated to be there, the person who is unwell may feel overwhelmed,
so visitors should take their cue from the patient. Similarly, "enemies" are discouraged from visiting (according to the rabbis,
"enemies" refers primarily to competitors in business and those who
might cause the patient anxiety). Visits during the first few days of
illness are reserved for family and close friends. However, if the illness comes suddenly, people should visit the patient immediately because of the life-threatening nature of the illness.

While we visit, we must be conscious of preserving the person's dignity. We should treat him or her just as we would in other
contexts. This is particularly true with regard to the laws and customs that regulate *tzniyut* (modesty). It is one of the reasons why
Jewish law advises against visiting during the first or last three
hours of the day, when a patient's personal needs are addressed. It
may also be that a patient requires a lot of assistance at the beginning of the day and feels worse toward the end of the day. As such,
the visitor is discouraged from presenting any sense of despair as
the condition appears to worsen. We are also taught not to visit
those who have intestinal problems in order to avoid embarrass-
ment, or those who are having certain pains (in the eye or head)
in order to prevent further pain or discomfort.

What to Do When You Visit

In addition to saying prayers of healing for the one who is ill (as
discussed in chapter 3), the essential obligation of the visitor is to

attend to that person's needs, to determine what needs to be done for his or her benefit, and to provide companionship, which emphasizes that he or she is not facing the illness alone. Moreover, each individual represents the community in order to affirm the same idea—we are not alone when we face illness. We face it as a community, just as we pray in the context of community.

According to the advice of those at the National Center for Jewish Healing, there are some specific behaviors that will enhance your visit. Allow the person to speak freely. Listen to him or her without scrutiny or judgment. Include reminders of his or her normative self and interests. Show concern and empathy. Be friendly and cheerful. Show respect for the person's human dignity. Be fully present. Avoid excessive references to the person's health unless initiated by the person who is ill. Don't bring outside concerns into the room. Avoid making excuses for not visiting sooner or more often. Do not offer medical advice. Don't attempt to "fix" the person's situation.

According to Rabbi Tsvi Blanchard, a faculty member of CLAL: National Jewish Center for Leadership and Learning, the sick bed is a matrix for holiness, just as the ancient Temple was, because God is present as a healer. We sit at the foot of the bed, avoiding any chair that is higher than the patient's to show that we are at the same level. The Talmud says that we should not sit at the head of the bed because the divine presence dwells there (*Shabbat* 12a). That is what makes *bikur cholim* an awesome experience—visiting the sick provides the possibility of experiencing the presence of God. The visitor is able to acknowledge the nurturing presence of God while simultaneously raising his or her own spirit. Rashi says that our posture is out of reverence for God's presence, which has descended in our midst to be with the sick patient.

Maimonides advises that the visitor should "wrap oneself up [that is, cloak oneself for a serious purpose] and sit below the head

of the bed and request divine mercy on [the patient's] behalf."
Speak honestly and directly while providing nurturance and support. Only answer questions that are asked, and avoid encourag-
ing both unrealistic hope and unnecessary despair.

Learning to Emulate God

The Talmud describes God's visit to Abraham following his cir-
cumcision (*Sotah* 14a). It is a simple act that we are instructed to
emulate. Other sources suggest that God sent an angel to bring divine healing to Abraham (Babylonian Talmud, *Bava Metzia* 86b).
We can be those angels and bring divine healing to those we love.

It is sometimes difficult for me to accept the responsibility
that I have as a channel for bringing God's healing into the world.
I feel it as a fellow human being and as a fellow Jew, and even
more so as a rabbi. Yet, I have felt the presence of God in the many
sick rooms I have visited, sometimes more profoundly than in any
other setting. And when I do, I know that I am a partner with
God in bringing healing.

Rabbi Hama son of Rabbi Hanina said, "What does the text
mean, 'you should walk after *Adonai* your God (Deuteronomy
13:5)'? Is it possible for a human being to walk after the *Shekhinah*
[divine presence]? Has it not also been said that '*Adonai* your God
is a devouring fire (Deuteronomy 4:24)'? The meaning is to walk
after (that is, to emulate) the attributes of the Holy One of
Blessing. As God clothes the naked, so you should clothe the
naked. As the Holy Blessed One visits the sick, so you should do
the same (Babylonian Talmud, *Sotah* 14a)." In the process of recovery, the human being is not only emulating God, but is also a
partner with God.

SIX

The Process of Recovery

Recovery is not a goal. It is a process that begins from the time you are diagnosed until the time you take your last breath on this earth (may it not be for many years). Like *teshuvah* (repentance), we may consider recovery a life-long process. Some even postulate that we begin our recovery at birth; in the womb, we are taught the entire Torah, only to be born and lose our Torah knowledge. It becomes a memory, a lost love to which we yearn to return. If the Torah provides a spiritual blueprint for healing, the moment we begin experiencing it, we are in recovery, and the process of healing begins. Because illness is something that presents us with a new prism through which to evaluate our lives, recovery is the process that affords us the opportunity to make changes. This process of recovery actually improves the quality of life, even if does not add years to it. Acknowledging the prospect of death is a transformative experience that can potentially get you on the road to recovery.

According to the rabbis, decisions about life and death are made by God each year during Yom Kippur. We influence this decision by our actions during the previous months. In the Jewish tradition, three factors mitigate the severity of the decision: *tefillah* (prayer), *tzedakah* (charity), and *teshuvah* (repentance). So we spend the month just prior to the fall holidays (Elul) reflecting on our lives and planning appropriate changes as we progress toward personal improvement. As we work through this process each year, we develop a posture for recovery from illness. Thus, recovery is an indigenous part of the Jewish calendar, built into it—for everyone—to ensure that we all have the correct tools when we have to use them. We are not forced to start from scratch when we are sick and most vulnerable.

For most people, illness and the process of recovery that is required of it presents the opportunity for a transformational experience. Others enact rituals that aid in this transformation. Some people either change their names or add additional ones. Men may become *Chaim,* women, *Chaya*. There are those who may regard this practice as primitive and superstitious, but such a name change can help individuals to redirect their lives in a profound way. They actually become another person. There are other turning points in life in which name changes might accomplish the same thing. When people immigrate to another country, they often take on a different name, as do many immigrants to the state of Israel. Any new name must be accompanied by a new mission and vision. This renewal of spirit is meant to speed the renewal of body.

Changing Perspectives

When my wife, Sheryl, was first diagnosed with cancer, we approached it as we did most other challenges in our lives. Perhaps it was my masculine approach to life, something that I had been socialized into, something that I did rather regularly no matter how banal or sublime the challenge. The cancer was a "problem" that required "fixing," so we sought out the appropriate means to fix it. In Sheryl's case, the course of action was primarily surgery as she was not a candidate for the radioactive iodine protocol. The surgeon assured us that once the cancer was surgically removed, she would not have to deal with it again and we could go on with our lives. Once we made it to the five-year mark, we would be "home free"; at that time, she would be considered in full remission. Sometimes consciously, sometimes unconsciously, we marked the time. We measured every occasion, whether it be a birthday, an anniversary, or even something simple like the beginning of the annual swim season at the local swim club, in relation to the surgery and the five-year mark. Sheryl and I seldom talked about the foundation of our calendric lives. We didn't have to.

We waited impatiently for five years to pass. We did what I have taught my children not to do: We lost the meaning of time by waiting for it to go by. Nevertheless, we even planned to celebrate Sheryl's five-year anniversary with a trip to the islands. As we approached the five-year mark, Sheryl's cancer reappeared, discovered during a routine exam by the doctor. Just as it had announced itself without warning the first time, it came back without warning, without any symptoms. All that waiting, all that anticipation appeared to be for naught. We thought we would have to start our countdown again. Five more years until we would be free. I wondered at the time whether the ancient Israelites felt the same way in the desert. As readers of the Torah, we know that they will ultimately be there for forty years, and we count down each episode as it is related in the biblical narrative. Were they feeling the same as we were?

"In the Thickness of a Dark Cloud"

Surgery was indicated once again, and this time it was to be much more extensive, more radical. After that hospitalization, we stopped counting the days and the weeks and the months and the years. We vowed not to live by this time clock. We knew that if we had to think ahead five more years, it would also be five years of our children's adolescent development that would be eclipsed and that, we reasoned, was a more important time clock. Though the teenage years are always trying, they are too precious to wish them forward too quickly. Instead, we decided that we would live with the disease as long as it was necessary. We knew that meant for the rest of our lives. We embraced it. Sheryl's struggle with cancer became part of who we were. By holding it close, we were able to wrestle its hold away from us. Like Jacob who wrestled with the stranger throughout the night and did not understand the presence of God until the darkness was obliterated by the light, we arrived at the same understanding. When finally Jacob let go of the stranger in the night and forced his opponent to bless him, Jacob emerged in the midst of the blessing with a new name: Israel—someone who struggled and triumphed. Jacob/Israel did not leave the encounter with "the other" without injury; that injury marked him the rest of his life. He paid a price for that blessing. So did we, but we felt blessed nonetheless.

Rabbi David Moshe of Tchortkov, one of my favorite teachers in Jewish tradition, said that the presence of God is often contained in the thickness of darkness. Although the world is full of the glory of God, the divine presence is accentuated in the darkness of distress. Moses knew where to approach God; "in the thickness of a dark cloud" (Exodus 19:9). And that is where Moses was able to most profoundly experience God's presence. In the darkness of illness and its aftermath, we experience God in ways that are previously unimaginable. It was in the darkness of Sheryl's illness that our relationship found the brightest light, a reflection of the divine light that we had let into our lives.

We integrated Sheryl's recovery into our lives. We learned to live with her cancer as a "chronic illness" even though there were no remaining signs of its presence. Trips to the doctor for routine examinations and to the hospital for tests and evaluation no longer frightened us. They became as much a part of our routine as anything else. They entered into the rhythm of our lives. We knew full well that if, God forbid, the cancer resurfaced, we would confront that challenge as we had before. We refused to allow it to control our lives. The rabbis were right when they wrote, "One cannot fully understand Torah unless one stumbles in it" (Babylonian Talmud, *Gittin* 43a).

Changing Directions

Our direct encounter with the angel of death on at least two separate occasions—although that dark angel hovers near us at various other times, as well—forced us to reconsider all of our relationships. Acquaintances and shallow relationships no longer seemed relevant. We spent time with friends whom we considered part of our extended family. Each moment we spent with our children, with members of our family, and with each other was considered a gift and we cherished it as such.

It also forced us to reevaluate what we were doing with our lives, and within the context of our family life. We recalled and implemented agreements that we had made earlier in our lives as we started our new family, things we had since forgotten. First, no one went to sleep angry. Second, no one left the house with unresolved conflicts or anger; we always wanted to ensure that potential last moments were lasting memories. Most of all, as Shabbat cast its brilliant shadow each week in our home, we made a contract that even when we might have a disagreement (something not unusual when trying to raise two fiercely independent adolescents), everything would be set aside at Shabbat. Just as *kiddush* helped us consecrate the day and make the distinction between the days of the workweek and the sacred timelessness of Shabbat, we made the distinction between petty everyday arguments and the possibilities in relationships that we could only imagine in the unique atmosphere of Shabbat. We believed that this was part of our family's journey toward building a religious life and we also recognized that this was all part of our recovery process. Shabbat helped us to heal, just as it had our people for many years before us. For that period of time we could return to Eden, we could get a glimpse of the world-to-come. In neither place is there suffering or pain.

That was our approach. Though we may talk about survival and recovery as if they are similar for everyone regardless of the physical challenges they face or the illness that caused their struggle, different people react to the same disease in very different ways. Treatments don't impact on everyone the same way. The road to recovery likewise takes people on disparate journeys. People perceive the messages of illness differently. One person told me that she considers angels to be directly related to the inner strength she must constantly garner in her struggle with disease. She believes that God sends angels to her in various forms to remind her that she has to muster the strength to regain control of her health, to tell her that her destiny is in her hands. These divine emissaries whisper to her, "Don't forget. There are other paths to take in life besides work." Just as we have come to understand that the path toward a religious life is ongoing, so is the process of recovery. We are never fully recovered. We take the journey step by step, day by day.

Living in the Moment

Illness is a powerful and influential teacher, but you have to be willing to learn. Like any good teacher, illness impacts on many people, not just on those who are sick. As we have discovered, illness teaches us many things including the essential focus of Jewish life: living in the moment. Although our tradition goes out of its way to honor memory and takes pains to ensure that we plan for the future, the most important moment is now, as we live it. We recall the path our people has taken. We mark sacred time and sacred place. But today must be our focus. If we dwell on the past or worry too much about the future, we may lose the present.

Rabbi Nachman of Breslov taught, "Think only about today. Think only about the present day and the present moment. When someone wants to start serving God, it seems too much of a burden to bear. But if you remember that you only have today, it won't be such a burden. Don't put off serving God from one day to the next, saying, 'I'll start tomorrow—tomorrow I'll pray with proper concentration.' All a person has is the present day and the present moment. Tomorrow is a whole different world." (*Likutey Moharan* I 272).

In the liturgy for Rosh Hashanah, the holiday said to mark the creation of the world, there is emphasis on one well-known prayer, *Hayom* (today). To stress this idea, the word is repeated over and over, particularly in the lilting mode of prayer chants.

The Torah tells us to choose life *today*. It offers us no other real option.

Surviving Cancer

People do not always survive cancer. It is part of the reality I face in the healing work I do. However, no one is in a position to determine how long a person has to live. Too often people give up because they are told they are "terminal." "We make our own miracles," one patient told me and continues to survive well beyond the limited years that were conjectured to her by her physician. Too many people leave it all to the medicines and the physicians and neglect the work toward healing that they have to do.

"Cancer has real Torah to teach," one patient reminded me. It taught him about the miracles of deliverance and redemption.

It taught him about the desert journey. It taught him about the essence of life and what is really important in it. As a result of his "education," he led a new life.

Battling Addictions and Compulsive Behaviors

There is a whole range of chemical addictions and compulsive behaviors with which people struggle. Their journey to recovery usually includes battling long-term abuse of a particular substance or behavior. What often leads people to seek help in battling their addictions is what is known as "bottoming out," an often near-death experience in which a person realizes that he or she can get no lower. Even so, it often takes an intervention by a "team" that includes family members to help the person realize that he or she has hit bottom.

Recovery is not a straight line from one place to another. Relapses are part of the path of recovery for most people. In the case of chemical addiction, this process begins with cleansing the body of its poisons: the addict's chemical of choice. Next, a change in the pattern of behaviors that are associated with the addiction, or which provide the context for the compulsive behavior. Along the way, addicts have to probe the depths of their souls in order to understand why they were "using" in the first place. This therapeutic process of introspection is tied to issues of self-esteem. Addicts frequently feel like there is a hole inside of themselves that they try to fill up with chemicals or food. They want to deaden the feeling of worthlessness with chemicals or with the high they get from compulsive gambling. They confuse sex with love because they feel so unloved. Above all, they feel alone. As part of the recovery process, addicts are helped to enter the covenantal relationship with God so that they come to understand that they are never alone.

I am not a faith healer. However, I have been changed through the experience of healing. When I visited Joshua, a former congregant, in his hospital room, his wife was sitting by his bed. She was fighting a drug addiction and Josh was very worried about her, terrified about what would become of her if he were to die. I took his hand in mine. He, in turn, took his wife's hand. And we prayed. A certain presence swept over us. I felt certain that Joshua would return to health, but he died. However, after that moment in the hospital room, his wife fought her addiction from a new direction and with a resolve that I had never before witnessed. In the midst of our prayers, she was healed.

Changing Approaches

Recounting his own experience with illness, Rabbi William Cutter, who writes extensively on healing and hospice, advises patients to write about their illnesses or at least find the proper figures of speech to describe them. This articulation helps people gain control of their illnesses, and find concrete expression for the potential emptiness that lies behind every disease. If one does not find a way to deal with the emptiness, healing is elusive. The soul may suffer while being severely diminished.

Journaling

Some people are predisposed to writing down events of the day—either as a way of planning events, perhaps in a daily organizer, or as a reflection after the events, as in a diary or journal. Others need inspiration and guidance to jot down even a few words. At various times in the Jewish calendar year, our tradition suggests that we reflect on our experiences in an effort to grow from them, using specific texts to help us gain insight (such as is the case with Psalm 27 during the month of Elul, the month preceding Rosh

Hashanah). Because reading and writing about experiences help people reflect on them, keeping a journal as a record of illness is an important part of the recovery process. Journal writing helps people identify and explore each feeling, each new insight, everything they learned as a result of the illness. Journaling also helps with the important task of detailing their progress—even when that progress is slight and nearly imperceptible. By putting things out on the table, we are able to see them more clearly.

Most women are more comfortable keeping journals than are their male counterparts. That's why it is even more important for men to do so. For men, the keeping of a journal that is not directed and has no specific template or predetermined paradigm helps them engage their recovery.

There are a variety of techniques that may be employed in the keeping of journals. I prefer to set aside a few minutes each day. Just as I say my morning prayers moments after I awaken and do exercises to strengthen my lower back prior to getting into bed at night, I have built a specific time of day into my routine for writing things down. It has become another part of my daily discipline. Thus, I have established a certain rhythm, a specific pattern for my writing. It makes the process a little easier—even though words do not always come when I want them.

Some people like to write down whatever comes to mind. I prefer to review the events of my day, the encounters with people, both positive and negative. Often physicians will ask a series of questions to plot the progress of recovery. These questions can also serve as guideposts in your journal because they often lead us to new discoveries about ourselves and the world around us.

The mystics in Safed used this technique each week as they ushered the Sabbath queen into their lives. As dusk descended upon them on Friday evening, they would walk up to the mountain peak in nearby Meron, and as they recited each psalm in the *Kabbalat Shabbat* service, they would review the events of the week. This helped them gain perspective prior to entering Shabbat.

Whatever your method, as you begin the process of using a journal it may be helpful to focus on one idea, one thought. Probe it. Reflect on it. Draw from it the lesson that will be helpful to your recovery.

Visualization

Visualizations are also helpful in the healing process and are very important to the process of recovery. They provide you with the state of mind that allows your body and spirit to be centered once again, to find *shelemut* (wholeness). While some visualizations are destructive and violent and may be useful in battling disease, I prefer those that are soothing and peaceful to aid recovery. They calm the spirit so that the body may heal.

On the Wings of Healing

Visualize God's ministering angels surrounding you. On your right is Michael, who offers you grace. On your left is Gabriel, who helps you regain strength. In front of you is Uriel, filled with soft light. And behind you is Raphael, who brings you continuous healing. All around you is the presence of *Shekhinah,* a loving God. As you become more comfortable with the process of visualization, you can focus your spiritual energy on any one of these angels, specifically for the resources each offers. From Michael, get love. From Gabriel, gain strength. From Uriel, receive the light of clarity and wisdom. And from Raphael, be healed. According to one midrash, when a parent puts a child to bed at night, God changes places with the child, allowing him or her to be protected by the very angels that minister to God all day long. Imagine yourself in that place as well.

The Essential Torah Story of Passover

The exodus from Egypt frames the core experience of the Jewish people. It has become the centerpiece of our shared historical memory. Because it details the triumphant deliverance from slavery to freedom, it has become *the* primary metaphor for liberation in the western world. Moreover, the account of Passover, the spring holiday which celebrates this journey from enslavement in Egypt to redemption in the promised land, presents the universal message of hope that informs the Jewish perspective on life. It can also provide us with the same unyielding message in the face of our recovery.

The annual recollection of this story each spring is incorporated as part of our ongoing process of recuperation. Imagine yourself leaving Egypt, leaving slavery behind It is the middle of the night and you must rush out. You choose only the things that are essential for your survival in the journey ahead of you. Although there are many people around you, you feel as if you are making the journey by yourself, utterly alone. The Egyptians are in hot pursuit. Finally, you reach the edge of the Red Sea. While others do not know what to do, you walk right in—and the waters part.

SEVEN

Waiting Until Messiah Comes or, At Least Until the Next Office Visit

There is a deeply moving, sentimental scene near the conclusion of the well-known movie *Fiddler on the Roof.* For many of us, it's reminiscent of what our grandparents went through when they were forced to leave their villages and *shtetlach* in Russia at the turn of the century. As the Jewish residents of fictional Anatevka prepare themselves to flee their hometown, one member of the community asks his rabbi about the Messiah. He remarks to the rabbi that the Jewish people has been waiting for the Messiah throughout a history of wandering. In the thick of their suffering, wouldn't now be a perfect time for his arrival? After a brief reflective pause, the rabbi—whose eyes brim with understanding—responds, "We'll just have to wait for him somewhere else." And so life goes on.

As we proceed on the path to personal healing, many of us think that it would be a good time for the Messiah to come. We pray for the Messiah's arrival each day in our formal prayers. Until the Messiah's arrival, we must persist in our full-time commitment to healing. This ongoing process places constant demands on us and on our families and friends. Everything else is second in priority to our healing. Our family has to realize that, as does our employer. And we have to hear ourselves saying it, as well. We will have to shift priorities in order to find the way to healing. And once we get on it, we cannot leave it. As a result of the disease we faced, we must be ever-vigilant. Every cough, sniffle, sneeze; every unusual rash, bump, or bruise gives us pause and demands scrutiny, definition, and diagnosis. Common little nuisances take on different proportions in our lives after we have confronted a life-threatening disease. The angel of death, even once defeated, continues a vigil in our midst. And so with each discomfort, we are returned to that place where we once were when we first encountered our illness. Even when it's only a momentary scare, it is as if the time that has passed has been eclipsed and we are back at the beginning of the process once again.

If we recognize that some diseases, like cancer, are ever-present in our bodies and rise to the surface when our immune systems are depressed, then we have to make permanent drastic changes in our lives in order to recover. This is the posture that should be maintained between our regular doctor visits as well. First, we must identify some of the factors that prevent our immune systems from fighting off a disease kept in abeyance for many years. Then we make the changes. These modifications have to be maintained even after we begin to feel like our original selves once again or we run the risk of returning to the place we were before we became sick. Recovery is maintained by some of the same approaches to a disciplined Jewish life that were proposed for healing and that got on us on the road to recovery in the first place: prayer, ritual, and study. Thus, visits to the physician should be complemented by visits to a rabbi whose talent for spiritual guidance has been demonstrated. This provides us with an environment in which to make sense out of our prayer, ritual, and study.

It must be emphasized that such an approach also helps the survivor to heal. Sometimes, the one we love is healed of soul but not of body. And so we turn to the rhythms of Jewish life to bring healing to the soul of the survivor.

Learning to Endure the Desert

After our people crossed the Red Sea from Egypt, they had to make their way through the desert. I wonder whether, after leaving Egypt, the Israelites had any idea of the real journey that lay ahead of them. Perhaps they thought they would simply make their way through the desert, a few weeks' trip at most. Yet, it took them forty years! Why did it take so long? It's clear from our reading of the Torah and our own experiences in the desert that such journeys of transformation take a long time. In the book of Exodus, God alludes to this when suggesting that divine guidance would lead the Jewish people the long way to the promised land instead of the most direct route.

Sometimes, the straightest route to healing takes us the long way around. Healing does not happen overnight, even when our disease is under control and no longer life-threatening. The desert journey of our people taught us how to endure the desert in life for an extended period of time. It is like spiritual DNA. Like the tablets of the covenant, which were said to be written with black fire on white fire, the journey of our people is written with spiritual fire on our genes. It is part of the Jewish religious psyche. It helps fuel the historical memory of the Jewish people. Now we add our personal journey to the collective one of our people. In doing so, our experience helps others face theirs. As fellow travelers, we make the spiritual trek together.

One of my favorite commentaries on understanding the challenges in life comes from the Talmud. It is a response to the question that we all ask: "When will the Messiah come?" Some perceive this as a question of theology. I have always read it as an expression of yearning for personal redemption—not "When will the world be saved?" but, "When will I be relieved of my suffering, when will this all be over?" People similarly misread liturgy all the time. They read the texts in the prayerbook and reject them because they do not seem to reflect their realities. However, the liturgy often paints a picture of a reality that can be brought into being, rather than one that already exists.

Hearkening to God's Voice

It seems that Rabbi Joshua ben Levi met the prophet Elijah (who, according to Jewish tradition, will announce the arrival of the Messiah) standing at the entrance to the cave of Rabbi Simon bar Yochai, to whom the central Jewish mystical text, the *Zohar,* is ascribed. Joshua asked Elijah when the Messiah would come. Elijah replied, "Go and ask him yourself."

"Where can I find him?" asked Joshua.

"Outside the gates of the city."

"And how will I recognize him?" asked Joshua.

Elijah responded, "He will be sitting among the poor people, covered with wounds. He and others unbind all the bandages on their wounds at once and then wrap them up again. Only the Messiah unbinds each of his wounds separately and then immediately covers them. He says to himself, 'If I am needed, I must be ready to go and not be late.'"

So Joshua went to the gates of the city and found him. "May peace be with you, my master and teacher."

He answered, "And may you be at peace, son of Levi."

Joshua continued the conversation, "When are you coming, master?" Immediately came the response, "Today."

So Joshua returned to Elijah and said, "He deceived me. He said that he would come today, but he has not come."

Elijah responded, "This is what he meant: 'Today—if you will hearken to God's voice' (Psalm 95:7)" (Babylonian Talmud, *Sanhedrin* 98a).

Perhaps it is true, that the messianic era will dawn *when* we have learned to hearken to God's voice. Illness is a challenge to live—differently. It provides us with the ultimate challenge to listen to God's voice in a way we might never have heard before. So turn your thoughts to God during each part of your treatment and afterwards.

Walking the Narrow Bridge

In order to accomplish this, as difficult as it may seem, follow this piece of advice of the rabbis, and "Repent a day before your death" (*Pirke Avot* 2:10), which means every day. Or as my friend Debbie Friedman puts it in her music, "Seize the moment. Seize the day." In their wisdom, the rabbis wanted us to keep our mortality forefront in our minds. Only when we understand death can we understand the sanctity of life. It is what drives us crazy sometimes about the behavior of adolescents. Too often they toy with life, thinking they are strong enough to overcome anything. The rabbis understood the spiritual logic implied in what they wrote in *Pirke Avot,* a book of wisdom on everyday life. They wanted to help direct the course of our lives, especially during illness and recovery. Their teachings echoed the sentiment of the prophet Isaiah, "The heart will understand. They will repent and be healed" (Isaiah 6:10).

The purpose of life is to come closer to God. Death— whether it comes sooner or later, and it will come eventually (but only to the body)—is the next stage of life. Confronting the possibility of corporeal death opens us up to an awesome experience with God, one that might not have taken place had illness not befallen us. The decision to live to the fullest, even with the limitations of illness, is a major step toward healing.

There is healing in peace, in the feeling of *shelemut* (wholeness) that accompanies recovery. We have to try to live without anxiety, without the disquieting anticipation of the next office visit. I have been told that waiting is the hardest part of illness. I know that it is true of our family. That's when the well-known words of Rabbi Nachman of Breslov come to mind, "*Kol ha-olam kulo gesher tzar me'od ve'ha-ikar lo lefached k'lal.* The whole world is a very narrow bridge. The essential thing is not to be afraid" (*Likutey Moharan* 2:28). Even when we are healed, when the cancer is in remission, when the disease leaves our body, we are still ill at ease. Every sniffle, every common flu or virus, causes us worry. And so we wait impatiently for the next routine doctor visit just to get reassurance.

But What Do We Do in the Meantime?

Follow the advice of the Torah: "Take care of yourself and treat your soul diligently" (Deuteronomy 4:9). Continue to pray. Continue to love. Continue to work. And continue to hope. There is a traditional framework for prayer that brings discipline in one's life. Each evening when I go to sleep, I look forward for the opportunity in the morning to get up and say my daily prayers and blessings. In the quiet of the house, I am aware of the same thing Jacob realized after he dreamed of a ladder stretching to heaven with angels ascending and descending. He reflected, "God was in this place and I certainly was not aware of it" (Genesis 28:16). Saying prayers in the morning hush of my house while the rest of my family sleeps, as the sun peeks through the windows and the birds chirp in the background, helps me remember that God is surely in this place and I feel the nurturing divine presence around me.

Love is reciprocal. The more we are willing to give, the more we are able to receive. Expressing love is not easy for some. For others, the words flow out without depth or meaning. God offers us a pattern of love and sustenance that should act as a model for our relationships with others.

Erich Fromm once wrote that love and work are the primary tasks in life, for they provide us with meaning and direction. When he spoke of work, he did not mean "get a job and make yourself useful." One of the challenges that comes to our attention during illness is to determine what our real work is in this world. What were we placed on this earth to accomplish? This becomes a main focus of our energy during office visits, and our attempt to bring Messiah: doing our intended work in the world. Often I joke that I try not to let my job get in the way of my work. Sometimes it's my job that allows me to do the work that I am meant to do.

Hope. It was Louis Brandeis who once reflected on the unusual ability of the Jewish people to have hope in the face of incredible odds. Many people dream, he said, but the Jewish people have the unique ability to realize their dreams. It is this perpetual optimism that has carried the Jewish people on its wings throughout our journey in history.

Leading a Jewish Life

It is not enough to follow the words of the prophet Micah who taught, "Do justice. Love mercy and walk humbly with God" (Micah 6:8). Our lives need structure and meaning—this comes through the discipline of living a Jewish life. This may sound like the knee-jerk company line, what you might expect to hear from a rabbi, the punchline in the sermon that every rabbi gives. But read these words carefully: I believe that Jewish living leads to personal redemption. And individual personal redemption ultimately leads to the redemption of the world. We bring it on, one person at a time. We have to start this process with ourselves; redemption just doesn't come on its own. We have to work toward it. When you engage a ritual, you are bringing yourself closer to God, but you must initiate it. We grow into patterns of observance. Our ritual life evolves over time. There are obstacles to overcome, but we soon recognize the spiritual path and get on it. Judaism makes it easier by giving us direction and by setting aside certain times that emphasize our spiritual work. It is said that all year long we go out looking for God, but during the High Holiday period, God comes looking for us.

Practical Suggestions

Those who have been ill have taught me many things and have shared with me many profound insights, echoing the optimism of Job: "Light will shine on your paths" (Job 22:28). Moreover, they have also shared practical suggestions about how they accomplished the everyday, the routine—"real life," as one friend likes to put it. The lessons are simple.

Laugh loud and long. "A happy heart is good for healing" (Proverbs 17:22).

Enjoy the warmth of relationships. Treasure even the tense moments with those you love, the difficulty of raising children. "And you who fear my name, the sun of righteousness will shine for you, with healing in its rays" (Malachi 3:20).

Put things into absolute perspective. When you do so, some things that once had meaning lose their significance.

Be kind and gentle.

Refuse to be a victim. Stand your ground "on the subway and on the street," as New Yorkers like to say.

Love more.

Studying Sacred Texts

Studying the sacred texts of our tradition can be helpful as it helps to maintain the dialogue between individuals and God. The Bible offers us testimony on God speaking directly to us, by saying: "I am God who heals you" (Exodus 15:26). Sacred texts provide us with maps for our spiritual journey in life. We become part of the text when we fully engage it. And when it is fully engaged, we can feel God's presence.

Rabbi David Moshe of Tchortikov was not a large man. Once, when a heavy Torah was being dedicated, he had to hold it in his arms for a long time. After a while, a friend who was much bigger than he asked him, "Do you want me to take it?" David Moshe replied, "No, the holy ark of the covenant was also very heavy. It was nearly impossible to lift. But once it was lifted, it carried the men who lifted it. Once you hold something holy, it is not heavy anymore." That's the way I feel about the Torah. When we raise it high after we have read from it in the synagogue (this is called *hagbah;* my kids call it "huggy bear" because that's what they like to do with the Torah, hug it close to them), it is because our study of it has lifted us up.

Telling Our Story to Others

We must use the tale of our illness to bring this blessing to others. It is what some have called the quest narrative or story. As one Jewish poet wrote: Our lives are scrolls. We write on them what we want remembered.

In fact, our lives are scrolls, no less sacred than the ones that recorded the words of the Torah. Like the Torah scroll itself, we raise up the Torah of our lives. It has something to teach, and because it is holy, it will carry us.

Finding the Strength to Handle the Wait

Like many others who have come before me, I have learned how to wait, often in anticipation of that awesome day when God's voice will be heard throughout the world. Come wait with me.

For me, the most powerful moment in worship takes place just at the end of the Torah service. We have all stood together once again at Sinai and it is time to return the Torah to the ark. It is time to return to "real time" and the real world. Just as the ark is closed, we sing out "Turn us, Adonai, back to You, and we will return. Renew our days as of old" (Lamentations 5:21). We want to return to the desert when life was simpler, when we knew promise lay in front of us, when the encounters with God were easily ascertained.

We have come to the painful realization that our so-called therapeutic culture has not been able to bring us the healing we seek. Let me end, therefore, as many worship services do, with the final words of *Adon Olam,* probably the most powerful line in the entire liturgy. In our daily liturgy, we often take for granted this resource for healing in the form of a prayer because it concludes the worship and because the melodies often employed do nothing to enhance its powerful spiritual message of healing. In some synagogues, people are already taking off their *tallitot* (prayer shawls) while the song is sung. In others, people are already walking out the door while the last strains—the most powerful message—are being sung. Listen to the last words of *Adon Olam.* Although they are merely printed words on a page, let the melody you may remember help you soar toward heaven.

Let these words frame your thoughts on healing:

B'yado afkid ruchi, be'eit ishan v'a-ira, v'im ruchi gevi-a-ti, Adonai li v'lo ira.

Into God's hands I entrust my spirit, when I sleep and when I wake; and with my spirit and my body also, as long as God is with me, I will not fear.

Prayers, Texts, and Resources for Healing

✴

Asher yatzar: An alternative version

Blessed are You, Shaddai, who has formed us in wisdom, and created within us the spark of life. Each cell does the work of its creator; each organ's existence is a tribute to God. If but one element of this wondrous structure were to fail in its task, we could not stand before You and give thanks for sustenance. Let us cherish this gift of flesh and blood, honoring it as God's creation. Blessed are You, our God, who performs miracles of creation and healing.[1]

A Prayer from Reb Noson

This prayer, by a famous student of Rabbi Nachman of Breslov, seeks to combine the elements of body and soul and can be used in addition to *Asher yatzar* and *Elohai neshama* or instead of them.

God, you are the unconditional healer. Arouse Your love for me and heal me. Remove all flaws and blemishes from my body, from my *nefesh*, from my *ruach*, and from my *neshamah*. Send complete healing to all those who are sick. Faithful, loving healer, who heals the broken-hearted and binds up their wounds: "Heal me, O God, and I will be healed. Save me and I will be saved for You, O God You are my healer." Let me be whole and perfect, free of all flaws and blemishes.

Let peace reign between my shoulder and my body. Let my body be sanctified and purified until it becomes united with the soul, willingly and with great joy. Let my body and soul unite in love and peace to do Your will sincerely until I attain complete inner harmony and am ready to arrange my prayer before You perfectly. Let my prayer rise before You like the incense and perfect sacrifices offered by those who are whole and perfect. Amen.

Adapted from The Fiftieth Gate, Likutey Tefilot, *Reb Noson's Prayer*

Daily blessings from When the Body Hurts, the Soul Still Longs to Sing

This is a creative set of morning blessings compiled by Rabbi Nancy Flam from a collection written by her students. They may be added to the morning blessings as they appear in the prayer book.

Blessed is our eternal God, Creator of the universe, who has allowed me to experience both great pleasure and the chance to learn of life, for the hope offered by this new day.

I awake in pain, misery, and utter confusion; but still I awake. My life is sacred. My life has purpose and my soul houses holy spirit. I pray for healing and to heal others. I gratefully acknowledge today with its infinite possibilities and opportunities. And let me say, Amen.

Blessed is the eternal one who gives me the ability to remember those blessings which are still mine to affirm and the strength to arise anew each day.

Blessed are You, spirit of life, who has the power to release me from life but sustains me for Your purpose. Give me the strength to accept this life until that purpose is fulfilled.

Dear God: Thanks for providing me with so many rich experiences and helping lead me down a path woven with loving friends and family. My fond and grateful memories sustain me during this difficult time. I never feel alone with Your guiding presence surrounding me.

Dear God, heal my spirit, salve my pain, help to make me whole again.

Bleassed are You, *mekor chayim* (source of life), who has given me consciousness once again. With each day of life may I continue the task of *tikkun olam* (perfecting/repairing the world) and take wonder and joy in the miracle of life.

Although I am ill and falling, and my body is frail, thank You for still allowing me to experience the wonder and sacredness of life on this earth.

This has become the well-known adaptation of the traditional prayer for healing found in many liberal synagogues in North America.

Mi Sheberakh

Music by Debbie Friedman
Lyrics by Debbie Friedman and Drorah Setel
(based on the traditional Jewish prayer for healing)
Mi sheberakh avotenyu
Mekor habrakha limoteynu
May the source of strength
Who blessed the ones before us
Help us find the courage
To make our lives a blessing.
And let us say: Amen.
Mi sheberakh imoteynu
Mekor habrakha lavotenyu
Bless those in need of healing
With *refuah shleima:*
The renewal of body,
The renewal of spirit.
And let us say: Amen.

This is a personal prayer for healing that is included in the Reform Movement's Liturgy for the home.

"In sickness I turn to You, O God, for comfort and help. Strengthen within me the wondrous power of healing that You implanted in your children. Guide my doctors and nurses that they may speed my recovery. Let my dear ones find comfort and courage in the knowledge that You are with us at all times, in sickness and in health. May my sickness not weaken my faith in You, nor diminish my love for others. From my illness may I gain a fuller sympathy for all who suffer. I praise you O God, the source of healing."[2]

A Prayer by Levi Yitzchak of Berditchev

This is a prayer by the well-known Hasidic master who was known for his strident position toward God, called in the Jewish tradition *chutzpah clappei malah* (*chutzpah* in the Face of Heaven).

I do not know how to ask You, Lord of the world, and even if I did know, I could not bear to do it. How could I venture to ask You why everything happens as it does, why we are driven from one exile into another, why our foes are allowed to torment us so. But in the Haggadah, the parent of the one "who does not yet know how to ask" is told "it is incumbent upon You to disclose it to the child." And, Lord of the world, am I not Your child? I do not ask You to reveal to me the secret of Your ways—I could not stand it! But show me one thing; show me what this very moment means to me, what it demands of me, what You, God, are telling me through my life at this moment. I do not ask You to tell me *why* I suffer, but only whether I suffer for your sake!

Rabbi Levi Yitzchak of Berditchev

Two Prayers from the Talmud
(adapted by Danny Siegel)

May it be Your will, O my God
    and God of my ancestors,
to grace our lives with love
    and a feeling for the intimacy of all humanity
and peace and friendship,
    and may all our days flourish because we are hopeful,
and may the borders of our lives overflow with students,
    and may we enjoy our reward in paradise.
Arrange things so that we will have good hearts
    and good friends,
and allow us to awaken with our appropriate yearnings fulfilled,
    and may You consider our wishes to be decent-and-good.

Rabbi Yochanan's prayer, Jerusalem Talmud, Berachot 4:2

May it be Your will, O our God,
that we be allowed to stand in places of astonishing light
and not in dark places,

and may our hearts know no pain,

and may our vision not be so clouded
that we would not see all the blessings of Life
that You have given us.

Rabbi Alexandrai's or Rav Himnuna's prayer, Berachot 17a

A Prayer by Rabbi Nachman of Breslov

This is Rabbi Nachman of Breslov's prayer. It has been rendered into a more popular form by contemporary singer Debbie Friedman; that version immediately follows.

Master of the universe, grant me the ability to be alone.
May it be my custom to go outdoors each day amongst the
trees and grasses, among all growing things, and there may
I be alone and enter into prayer, to talk to the one to whom
I belong.

You Are the One (Reb Nachman's Prayer)

Music by Debbie Friedman
Lyrics by Debbie Friedman, based on Reb Nachman's prayer

You are the One, for this I pray,
That I may have the strength to be alone.
To see the world, to stand among the trees,
And all the living things.
That I may stand alone and offer prayers and talk to You;
You are the one to whom I do belong.
And I'll sing my soul,
I'll sing my soul to You.
And give You all that's in my heart.

May all the foliage of the field,
All grasses, trees and plants,
Awaken at my coming, this I pray,
And send their life into my words of prayer.
So that my speech, my thoughts, my prayers
    will be made whole,
And through the spirit of all growing things.
And we know that everything is one,
Because we know that everything is You.

You are the One, for this I pray,
I ask You, God, to hear my words
That pour out from my heart; I stand before You;
I, like water, lift my hands to You in prayer.
And grant me strength, and grant me strength to stand alone.
You are the One to whom I do belong.
And I'll sing my soul, I'll sing my soul to You
And give You all that's in my heart.

You are the One, for this I pray,
And I'll sing my soul to You.

Refa na lah

When Miriam was sick, her brother Moses prayed: "*El na, refa na lah;* O God, heal her please." We pray for those who are now ill. We pray for those who are affected by illness, anguish, and pain. Grant courage to those whose bodies, holy proof of Your creative goodness, are invaded by illness and pain. Grant strength and compassion to families and friends who give their loving care and support and help them to overcome despair.

Grant wisdom to those who probe the deepest complexities of Your world as they labor in the search for treatments and cures. Grant clarity of vision and strength of purpose to the leaders of our institutions and our government. May they be moved to act with justice and compassion. Grant insight to us, so we may understand that whenever death comes, we must accept it—but that before it comes, we must resist it by cherishing our lives and making our lives worthy as long as we live.[3]

Birkat HaGomel

On recovering from illness, one should recite *Birkat HaGomel.* This corresponds to the thanksgiving offering that was made in Temple times by those who were spared from a life-threatening situation. According to Jewish law, it should be recited in front of a *minyan,* preferably within the presence of at least two Torah scholars and within three days of the event. Generally, it takes place during the Torah reading in a synagogue by a person honored with an *aliyah.*

re You, *Adonai* our God, Sovereign of the
who bestows on us things that we may not de-
who has bestowed goodness on me.
regation responds,
Amen. May the One who bestows goodness on you continue to bestow goodness on you forever.

Three Prayers

We Are Loved by an Unending Love

We are loved by an unending love,
We are embraced by arms that find us
even when we are hidden from ourselves.
We are touched by fingers that soothe us even when
We are too proud for soothing.
We are counseled by voices that guide us
even when we are too embittered to hear.
We are loved by an unending love.
We are supported by hands that uplift us
even in the midst of a fall.
We are urged on by eyes that meet us
even when we are too weak for meeting.
We are loved by an unending love.
Embraced, touched, soothed, and counseled . . .
Ours are the arms, the fingers, the voices;
ours are the hands, the eyes, the smiles;
We are loved by an unending love.

Rabbi Rami M. Shapiro

O my God
My soul's compassion
My heart's precious friend
I turn to You.

In the silence of my innermost being,
In the fragment of my yearned-for wholeness,
I hear whispers of Your presence —

Echoes of the past when You were with me
When I felt Your nearness
When together we walked —
When You held me close, embraced me in Your love,
laughed with me in my joy.
I yearn to hear You again.

In Your oneness, I find healing.
In the promise of Your love, I am soothed.
In Your wholeness, I too become whole again.

Please listen to my call —
help me find the words
help me find the strength within
help me shape my mouth, my voice, my heart
so that I can direct my spirit and find You in prayer
In words only my heart can speak
In songs only my soul can sing
Lifting my eyes and heart to You.

Adonai
s'fatai tiftach
open my lips, precious God,
so that I can speak with You again.

Rabbi Sheldon Zimmerman

When I am lonely
O Great and Glorious God —
when I am lonely
I imagine You to be
my favorite uncle,
lost when I was yet an infant.
Forgive me,
for I am weak.

O Great God —
when I create a sorrow
I think of You as a friend
telling tales of bears
and clever foxes,
singing stories and drying tears.
Forgive me,
I am human.

My Gracious God —
when I consider death
I call to mind a kid,
a cat, a dog, a stick,
unto the thousand eyes
of Your most certain angel —
and Your promises forever.
Love me, Lord;
I am a child.

Danny Siegel

I call upon the Source of Life,
the Power within and without,
the Power that makes for
Being and Nothingness,
joy and pain,
suffering and delight.

> I call upon You
> to calm my fearful soul
> to open me to the Wonder of Truth
> the transience of all things.

In Wonder was I conceived
and in Wonder have I found my being.
Thus, I call upon You,
the Source of Wonder,
to open my heart to healing.

> In You I discover the mystery of life
> and the necessity of death.

In You I see all things and their opposites
not as warring parties
but as partners in a dance
whose rhythm is none other than
the beating of my own soul.

> Denial may come,
> but so too will acceptance.
> Anger may come,
> but so too will calm.

I have bargained with my fears
and found them unwilling to compromise.
So now I turn to You,
to the wonder that is my true nature.

> I abandon the false notions of separateness
> and embrace the Unity
> that is my true reality.

I surrender
not to the inevitable
but to surprise,
for it is the impossible
that is life's most precious gift.

> My tears will pass
> and so will my laughter.
> But I will not be silenced,
> for I will sing the praises of wonder
> through sickness and health;
> knowing that in the end,
> this too shall pass.

Rabbi Rami M. Shapiro

Prayer Visualizations

Certain prayers lend themselves to visualization, a powerful tool on the path to healing. For example, the evening service contains a prayer called *Hashkivenu*. This prayer asks for God's protection from the many things that might potentially harm us. In vivid imagery, we ask God in this prayer "to spread over us a covering of peace, *sukkat shelomekha*." In reciting this prayer, we can visualize ourselves standing under God's *sukkah*, God's shelter. Like the *sukkah* that we build each fall, it seems flimsy yet somehow seems to stand up against the storms that threaten it. Elsewhere in the service, we ask that God protect us "*tachat kanfei haShekhinah*, under the wings of the Divine Presence." This is the place we long to be: sheltered under God's nurturing wings.

Healing Centers and Organizations

The National Center for Jewish Healing

850 Seventh Ave., Suite 1201, New York, NY 10019

Tel: (212) 399-2320

Fax: (212) 399-2475

Website: www.jbfcs.org

This is the umbrella organization for Jewish healing centers in communities throughout North America. It publishes a variety of resources, it sponsors workshops and conferences, and it offers training opportunities, particularly for rabbis, health care professionals, and others who work in the Jewish community.

Other healing centers in North America, listed by state and then metropolitan area, follow in alphabetical order (see p. 117 for Canada). New healing centers are continually being established; this list includes longstanding as well as newer centers. Check with the synagogues or hospitals in your community for other healing centers in your area.

Arizona

Phoenix

Shalom Center for Education, Healing and Growth

4645 E. Marilyn Rd., Phoenix, AZ 85032

Tel: (602) 971-1234

Fax: (602) 971-5909

E-mail: shalomcenter@templechai.com

California

Los Angeles

The Jewish Healing Center at Metivta

2001 S. Barrington Ave., Suite 106, Los Angeles, CA 90025

Tel: (310) 477-5370

Fax: (310) 477-7501

E-mail: metivta@metivta.org

Orange County

Jewish Healing Center of Orange County

250 E. Baker St., Suite G, Costa Mesa, CA 92626

Tel: (714) 445-4950

Fax: (714) 445-4960

E-mail: jfsocmroth@earthlink.net

San Diego

The Jewish Healing Center Jewish Family Service

3715 Sixth Ave., San Diego, CA 92103

Tel: (619) 291-0473

Fax: (619) 291-2419

E-mail: jfs-sd@email.msn.com

San Francisco

Bay Area Jewish Healing Center
3330 Geary Blvd., Third Floor West, San Francisco, CA 94118
Tel: (415) 750-4197
Fax: (415) 750-4115
E-mail: jewishhealing@mzhf.org

Colorado

Denver/Boulder

Rafael: Jewish Spiritual Healing Center of Colorado
1355 S. Colorado Blvd., Denver, CO 80222
Tel: (303) 759-5199, x351 (Denver)
Tel: (303) 530-5494 (Boulder)

Delaware

Kimmel-Spiller Jewish Healing Center Jewish Family Service
101 Garden of Eden Rd., Wilmington, DE 19803
Tel: (302) 478-9411
Fax: (302) 479-9883
E-mail: klotzstein@aol.com

Washington, DC

Washington Jewish Healing Network
4707 Connecticut Ave. NW, Suite 104, Washington, DC 20008
Tel: (202) 966-7851
Fax: (202) 966-5422
E-mail: washheal@aol.com

Florida

Tampa

The Jewish Healing Center (of Tampa Jewish Family Service)
13009 Community Campus Dr., Tampa, FL 33625
Tel: (813) 960-1848
Fax: (813) 265-8239
E-mail: tjfs@gte.net

Maryland

Baltimore

Baltimore Jewish Healing Network
5750 Park Heights Ave., Baltimore, MD 21215
Tel: (410) 466-9200, ext. 110

Massachusetts

Boston

Jewish Healing Connections
(a service of Jewish Family and Children's Service)
1340 Centre St., Newton Centre, MA 02459
Tel: (617) 558-1278
Fax: (617) 559-5250
E-mail: msokoll@jfcsboston.org

Framingham

Healing Partners (a Jewish Family Service of Metrowest)
475 Franklin St., Suite 101, Framingham, MA 01702
Tel: (508) 875-3100
Fax: (508) 875-4373
E-mail: myoung@jfsmw.org

Minnesota
Minneapolis-St. Paul

Twin Cities Jewish Healing Program
(a service of Jewish Family and Children's Service)
13100 Wayzata Blvd., Suite 400, Minnetonka, MN 55305
Tel: (612) 542-4814
Fax: (612) 593-1778
E-mail: dlevenstein@jfcsmpls.org

Missouri
St. Louis

Jewish Family and Children's Service
(in cooperation with Congregation Shaare Emeth)
9385 Olive Blvd., St. Louis, MO 63132
Tel: (314) 993-1240

New Jersey
Clifton

Jewish Family Service of Clifton
199 Scoles Ave., Clifton, NJ 07012
Tel: (973) 777-7638
Fax: (973) 777-6701
E-mail: jfs1@jfedcliftonpossaic.com

Ventnor

The Jewish Healing Center of the Jewish Family Service
of Atlantic County
3 S. Weymouth Ave., Ventnor, NJ 08406
Tel: (609) 822-1108
Fax: (609) 822-1106
E-mail: jewishhealingcenter@jfsatlantic.org

New York

Hudson Valley

Jewish Family Services of Orange County

92 Seward Ave., Suite 7, Middletown, NY 10940

Tel: (914) 341-1173

New York City

New York Jewish Healing Center

(a Jewish Connections Program of the Jewish Board of Family

and Children's Services)

850 Seventh Ave., Suite 1201, New York, NY 10019

Tel: (212) 399-2320

Fax: (212) 399-2475

E-mail: jsherman@jbfcs.org

Rochester

Jewish Family Service

441 East Ave., Rochester, NY 14607

Tel: (716) 461-0110

Ohio

Cleveland

Cleveland Jewish Healing Center

1976 Temblethurst, South Euclid, OH 44121

Tel: (216) 381-6119

Pennsylvania

Allentown

Jewish Family Service of the Lehigh Valley
1136 Hamilton St., Suite 101, Allentown, PA 18101
Tel: (610) 821-8722
Fax: (610) 821-8925
E-mail: jfsoflv@enter.net

Harrisburg

The Jewish Healing Center of Harrisburg Jewish Family Service
3333 N. Front St., Harrisburg, PA 17110
Tel: (717) 233-1681
Fax: (717) 234-8258
E-mail: helecohen@aol.com

Pittsburgh

Shalom Network
6415 Monitor St., Pittsburgh, PA 15217
Tel: (412) 421-6912
Fax: (412) 648-6871
E-mail: gabrams18@aol.com

Canada

Toronto, Ontario

The Toronto Jewish Healing Project
603-55 Wellesley St. E.
Toronto, Ontario M4Y 2T6
Canada
Tel: (416) 944-3359
Fax: (416) 968-1996
E-mail: etta2000@sympatico.ca

Suggestions for Further Reading

Bleich, J. David. *Judaism and Healing: A Halakhic Perspective.* Hoboken, N.J.: KTAV, 1981.

This volume provides a straightforward legal treatment of sacred texts related to healing and health-related matters, written from the perspective of traditional Judaism.

Brenner, Daniel. *R'fuah: A Guide to Jewish Healing.* New York: CLAL—the National Jewish Center for Learning and Leadership, 1999.

This is an attractive, small volume that is very useful. It contains short prayers, texts, and source materials designed to be used for situations that require healing.

Cardin, Nina Beth. *Tears of Sorrow, Seeds of Hope: A Jewish Spiritual Companion for Infertility and Pregnancy Loss.* Woodstock, Vt.: Jewish Lights Publishing, 1999.

This is a spiritual companion for couples who have sought a Jewish expression for the pain they may have experienced following a lost pregnancy or while facing the challenges of infertility.

Finkel, Avraham Yakov. *In My Flesh I See God.* Northvale, N.J.: Jason Aronson, 1995.

This is an old text that has been recently reissued. It takes the form of an encyclopedia and extensively lists sacred Jewish texts that have to do with all aspects of the body and its function.

Flam, Nancy. *When the Body Hurts, the Soul Still Longs to Sing.* New York: National Center for Jewish Healing, 1992.

In the tradition of women's prayers, known as *tkhines,* this is a collection of prayers written by women who long to offer others spiritual uplift out of the midst of their experiences.

Freeman, David L., and Judith Z. Abrams, eds. *Illness and Healing in the Jewish Tradition.* Philadelphia: Jewish Publication Society of America, 1999.

Edited by a physician and a rabbi, this book is a treasure of resources from Jewish sources throughout history. It provides the reader with texts for any occasion or situation, as well as some guidance from the editors on the use of these resources.

Goldhamer, Douglas, and Melinda Stengel. *This Is for Everyone: Universal Principles of Healing Prayer and the Jewish Mystics.* Burdett, N.Y.: Larson Publications, 1998.

Following a step-by-step method, the authors introduce readers to the universal principles of healing embedded in Jewish mysticism. The book contains both a theoretical approach and practical exercises.

Greenbaum, Avraham. *Wings of the Sun: Traditional Jewish Healing in Theory and Practice.* Jerusalem: Breslov Research Institute, 1995.

Expanding on the teachings of Rabbi Nachman of Breslov, this book is rich in resource, insight, and inspiration. The author takes the reader through Rabbi Nachman's teachings as they relate to traditional perspectives on healing in the Jewish tradition.

―――. *A Call to Live: Jewish Guidance on Healing.* Jerusalem: Azamra Institute, 1999.

This is an insightful on-line book full of profound resources for those who are facing serious illness. Along with other resources for the journey of healing through Judaism, it is available at www.Azamra.org.

Jaffe, Hirschel, and H. Leonard Poller, eds. *Gates of Healing: A Message of Comfort and Hope.* New York: Central Conference of American Rabbis, 1991.

A small, pamphlet-sized collection of prayers, meditations, and readings to bring comfort, hope, and consolation to those who are ill, as well as those who care about them.

Nachman of Breslov. *The Empty Chair: Timeless Wisdom from a Hasidic Master, Rebbe Nachman of Breslov.* Adapted by Moshe Mykoff and the Breslov Research Institute. Woodstock, Vt.: Jewish Lights Publishing, 1994.

This is a wonderful collection of some of Rebbe Nachman of Breslov's most profoundly spiritual aphorisms. Each one offers insight and support to individuals as they navigate their way through life.

————. *The Gentle Weapon: Prayers for Everyday and Not-So-Everyday Moments—Timeless Wisdom from the Teachings of the Hasidic Master, Rebbe Nachman of Breslov.* Adapted by Moshe Mykoff and S. C. Mizrahi, together with the Breslov Research Institute. Woodstock, Vt.: Jewish Lights Publishing, 1999.

This is a treasure-trove of prayers that will open the heart, mind, and soul. In this little volume, Rabbi Nachman gives voice to our own most profound yearnings.

Polish, Daniel F. *Bringing the Psalms to Life: How to Understand and Use the Book of Psalms.* Woodstock, Vt.: Jewish Lights Publishing, 2000.

This book is an inspirational guidebook for all those who want to use the psalms to enhance their lives, particularly when facing spiritual challenges such as feeling abandoned, overcoming physical illness, addressing anger, and giving thanks. Rabbi Polish also presents readers with an overview of the textual tradition surrounding the psalms.

Polsky, Howard. *Everyday Miracles: The Healing Wisdom of Hasidic Stories.* Northvale, N.J.: Jason Aronson, 1989.

This is a collection of inspirational and unusual stories upon which the reader is invited to reflect.

Rosman, Steven. *Jewish Healing Wisdom.* Northvale N.J.: Jason Aronson, 1997.

This small volume provides the reader with a variety of sacred texts that span a wide range of Jewish themes, organized by subject area, without any narrative. Thus, it permits the individual to choose texts and apply them to his or her journey to healing as needed.

Schwartz, Dannel I., with Mark Hass. *Finding Joy: A Practical Spiritual Guide to Happiness.* Woodstock, Vt.: Jewish Lights Publishing, 1996.

This is a practical, how-to book for everyone who seeks happiness in their lives. And who doesn't? The book is based on the teachings of Jewish mysticism and the sacred texts of kabbalah.

Weintraub, Simkha Y., ed. *Healing of Soul, Healing of Body: Spiritual Leaders Unfold the Strength and Solace in Psalms.* Woodstock, Vt.: Jewish Lights Publishing, 1994.

This book features an inspiring translation of Rabbi Nachman of Breslov's collection of healing psalms (what he called a *tikkun klali*) with commentary by a group of rabbis and teachers who represent a wide spectrum of North American Jewry.

Wittenberg, Jonathan. *With Healing on Its Wings: Contemplations in Time of Illness.* London: Masorti Publications, n.d.

Text selections from a variety of traditional and contemporary sources that have been integrated into standard liturgies. In addition, the editor has included select prayers for situations such as before an operation and on recovering from illness.

Wolpe, David. *Making Loss Matter: Creating Meaning in Difficult Times.* New York: Riverhead Books, 1999.

"Losses are the stuff of life. They will not miss you, they will not steer around those whom you love." This is what author Rabbi David Wolpe says. Admittedly, his life became "full of shadows," a result of the fear that surfaced after his wife was diagnosed with cancer. He was afraid that she might die. Her illness gave him a new perspective on suffering. Although the book contains no new ideas or resources, you will want Rabbi Wolpe's sensitive insights to accompany you as you make your way through the desert.

Notes

Chapter 1

1. "The Death of a Child," CCAR source book on healing (n.p., n.d.).
2. Lawrence Kushner, *The Book of Words* (Woodstock Vt.: Jewish Lights Publishing, 1993), 48.
3. Ibid., 101.

Chapter 3

1. Abraham Joshua Heschel, "The Patient as a Person," *The Insecurity of Freedom: Essays on Human Existence* (New York: Farrar, Straus & Giroux, 1966), 255.
2. Martin Buber, *Tales of the Hasidim: Later Masters,* translated by Olga Marx (New York: Schocken Books, 1948), 90.
3. *A Leaders Guide to Services and Prayers of Healing* (New York: National Center for Jewish Healing, 1998).
4. "Sabbath Week," *The (New York) Jewish Week,* 28 May 1999.

Prayers, Texts, and Resources for Healing

1. *Machzor U'becharta Chayim,* Congregation Sha'ar Zahav, San Francisco, Calif.

2. Chaim Stern, ed. *On the Doorposts of Your House.* (New York: Central Conference of American Rabbis, 1995), 153.

3. *Refa na lah,* Congregation Sha'ar Zahav, San Francisco, Calif.

About JEWISH LIGHTS Publishing

People of all faiths and backgrounds yearn for books that attract, engage, educate and spiritually inspire.

Our principal goal is to stimulate thought and help all people learn about who the Jewish People are, where they come from, and what the future can be made to hold. While people of our diverse Jewish heritage are the primary audience, our books speak to people in the Christian world as well and will broaden their understanding of Judaism and the roots of their own faith.

We bring to you authors who are at the forefront of spiritual thought and experience. While each has something different to say, they all say it in a voice that you can hear.

Our books are designed to welcome you and then to engage, stimulate and inspire. We judge our success not only by whether or not our books are beautiful and commercially successful, but by whether or not they make a difference in your life.

We at Jewish Lights take great care to produce beautiful books that present meaningful spiritual content in a form that reflects the art of making high quality books. Therefore, we want to acknowledge those who contributed to the production of this book.

Stuart M. Matlins, Publisher

PRODUCTION
Marian B. Wallace & Bridgett Taylor

EDITORIAL
Sandra Korinchak, Emily Wichland,
Martha McKinney & Amanda Dupuis

JACKET DESIGN
Drena Fagen, New York, New York

TEXT DESIGN & TYPESETTING
Sans Serif, Inc., Saline, Michigan

COVER PRINTING
Pompy Press, East Thetford, Vermont

TEXT PRINTING AND BINDING
Edwards Brothers, Lillington, North Carolina

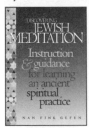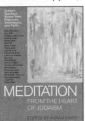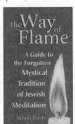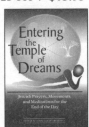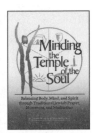

Spirituality

My People's Prayer Book: *Traditional Prayers, Modern Commentaries*

Ed. by *Dr. Lawrence A. Hoffman*

This momentous, critically-acclaimed series is truly a people's prayer book, one that provides a diverse and exciting commentary to the traditional liturgy. It will help modern men and women find new wisdom and guidance in Jewish prayer, and bring liturgy into their lives. Each book includes Hebrew text, modern translation, and commentaries *from all perspectives* of the Jewish world. Vol. 1—*The Sh'ma and Its Blessings*, 7 x 10, 168 pp, HC, ISBN 1-879045-79-6 **$23.95**
Vol. 2—*The Amidah*, 7 x 10, 240 pp, HC, ISBN 1-879045-80-X **$23.95**
Vol. 3—*P'sukei D'zimrah* (Morning Psalms), 7 x 10, 240 pp, HC, ISBN 1-879045-81-8 **$23.95**
Vol. 4—*Seder K'riyat Hatorah* (Shabbat Torah Service), 7 x 10, 240 pp, ISBN 1-879045-82-6 **$23.95**
(Avail. Sept. 2000)

Voices from Genesis: *Guiding Us through the Stages of Life*

by *Dr. Norman J. Cohen*

In a brilliant blending of modern *midrash* (finding contemporary meaning from biblical texts) and the life stages of Erik Erikson's developmental psychology, the characters of Genesis come alive to give us insights for our own journeys. 6 x 9, 192 pp, HC, ISBN 1-879045-75-3 **$21.95**

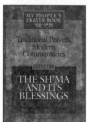 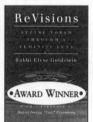 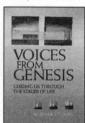 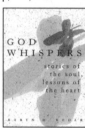 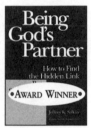

God Whispers: *Stories of the Soul, Lessons of the Heart*
by Rabbi Karyn D. Kedar 6 x 9, 176 pp, Quality PB, ISBN 1-58023-088-1 **$15.95**;
HC, ISBN 1-58023-023-7 **$19.95**

Being God's Partner: *How to Find the Hidden Link Between Spirituality and Your Work*
by Rabbi Jeffrey K. Salkin; Intro. by Norman Lear **AWARD WINNER!**
6 x 9, 192 pp, Quality PB, ISBN 1-879045-65-6 **$16.95**; HC, ISBN 1-879045-37-0 **$19.95**

ReVisions: *Seeing Torah through a Feminist Lens* **AWARD WINNER!**
by Rabbi Elyse Goldstein 5½ x 8½, 208 pp, HC, ISBN 1-58023-047-4 **$19.95**

Soul Judaism: *Dancing with God into a New Era*
by Rabbi Wayne Dosick 5½ x 8½, 304 pp, Quality PB, ISBN 1-58023-053-9 **$16.95**

Finding Joy: *A Practical Spiritual Guide to Happiness* **AWARD WINNER!**
by Rabbi Dannel I. Schwartz with Mark Hass
6 x 9, 192 pp, Quality PB, ISBN 1-58023-009-1 **$14.95**; HC, ISBN 1-879045-53-2 **$19.95**

The Empty Chair: *Finding Hope and Joy—*
Timeless Wisdom from a Hasidic Master, Rebbe Nachman of Breslov **AWARD WINNER!**
Adapted by Moshe Mykoff and the Breslov Research Institute
4 x 6, 128 pp, Deluxe PB, 2-color text, ISBN 1-879045-67-2 **$9.95**

The Gentle Weapon: *Prayers for Everyday and Not-So-Everyday Moments*
Adapted from the Wisdom of Rebbe Nachman of Breslov by Moshe Mykoff and
S. C. Mizrahi, with the Breslov Research Institute
4 x 6, 144 pp, Deluxe PB, 2-color text, ISBN 1-58023-022-9 **$9.95**

"Who Is a Jew?" *Conversations, Not Conclusions* by Meryl Hyman
6 x 9, 272 pp, Quality PB, ISBN 1-58023-052-0 **$16.95**; HC, ISBN 1-879045-76-1 **$23.95**

The Way Into... Series

A major 14-volume series to be completed over the next several years, *The Way Into...* provides an accessible and usable "guided tour" of the Jewish faith, its people, its history and beliefs—in total, an introduction to Judaism for adults that will enable them to understand and interact with sacred texts.

Each volume is written by a major modern scholar and teacher, and is organized around an important concept of Judaism.

The Way Into... will enable all readers to achieve a real sense of Jewish cultural literacy through guided study. Forthcoming volumes include:

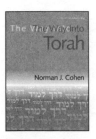
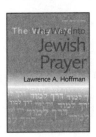
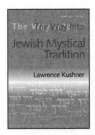
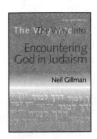

The Way Into Torah

by *Dr. Norman J. Cohen*

What is "Torah"? What are the different approaches to studying Torah? What are the different levels of understanding Torah? For whom is the study intended? Explores the origins and development of Torah, why it should be studied and how to do it. Addresses these and many other issues in this easy-to-use, easy-to-understand introduction to the ancient subject.

6 x 9, 160 pp, HC, ISBN 1-58023-028-8 **$21.95**

The Way Into Jewish Prayer

by *Dr. Lawrence A. Hoffman*

Explores the reasons for and the ways of Jewish prayer. Opens the door to 3,000 years of the Jewish way to God by making available all you need to feel at home in Jewish worship. Provides basic definitions of the terms you need to know as well as thoughtful analysis of the depth that lies beneath Jewish prayer.

6 x 9, 160 pp, HC, ISBN 1-58023-027-X **$21.95**

The Way Into Jewish Mystical Tradition

by *Rabbi Lawrence Kushner*

Explains the principles of Jewish mystical thinking, their religious and spiritual significance, and how they relate to our lives. A book that allows us to experience and understand the Jewish mystical approach to our place in the world.

6 x 9, 176 pp, HC, ISBN 1-58023-029-6 **$21.95** (Avail. Nov. 2000)

The Way Into Encountering God in Judaism

by *Dr. Neil Gillman*

Explains how Jews have encountered God throughout history—and today—by exploring the many metaphors for God in Jewish tradition. Explores the Jewish tradition's passionate but also conflicting ways of relating to God as Creator, relational partner, and a force in history and nature.

6 x 9, 176 pp, HC, ISBN 1-58023-025-3 **$21.95** (Avail. Nov. 2000)

Spirituality—The Kushner Series

Honey from the Rock, Special Anniversary Edition
An Introduction to Jewish Mysticism
by *Lawrence Kushner*

An insightful and absorbing introduction to the ten gates of Jewish mysticism and how it applies to daily life. "The easiest introduction to Jewish mysticism you can read."
6 x 9, 176 pp, Quality PB, ISBN 1-58023-073-3 **$15.95**

Eyes Remade for Wonder
The Way of Jewish Mysticism and Sacred Living
A Lawrence Kushner Reader

Intro. by *Thomas Moore*

Whether you are new to Kushner or a devoted fan, you'll find inspiration here. With samplings from each of Kushner's works, and a generous amount of new material, this book is to be read and reread, each time discovering deeper layers of meaning in our lives.
6 x 9, 240 pp, Quality PB, ISBN 1-58023-042-3 **$16.95**; HC, ISBN 1-58023-014-8 **$23.95**

Invisible Lines of Connection
Sacred Stories of the Ordinary
by *Lawrence Kushner* AWARD WINNER!

Through his everyday encounters with family, friends, colleagues and strangers, Kushner takes us deeply into our lives, finding flashes of spiritual insight in the process.
6 x 9, 160 pp, Quality PB, ISBN 1-879045-98-2 **$15.95**; HC, ISBN 1-879045-52-4 **$21.95**

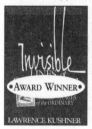 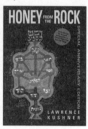 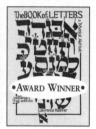 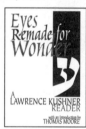 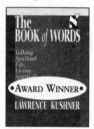

The Book of Letters
A Mystical Hebrew Alphabet AWARD WINNER!
by Lawrence Kushner
Popular HC Edition, 6 x 9, 80 pp, 2-color text, ISBN 1-879045-00-1 **$24.95**; *Deluxe Gift Edition*, 9 x 12, 80 pp, HC, 2-color text, ornamentation, slipcase, ISBN 1-879045-01-X **$79.95**; *Collector's Limited Edition*, 9 x 12, 80 pp, HC, gold-embossed pages, hand-assembled slipcase. With silkscreened print. Limited to 500 signed and numbered copies, ISBN 1-879045-04-4 **$349.00**

The Book of Words
Talking Spiritual Life, Living Spiritual Talk AWARD WINNER!
by Lawrence Kushner 6 x 9, 160 pp, Quality PB, 2-color text, ISBN 1-58023-020-2 **$16.95**; 152 pp, HC, ISBN 1-879045-35-4 **$21.95**

God Was in This Place & I, i Did Not Know
Finding Self, Spirituality & Ultimate Meaning
by Lawrence Kushner 6 x 9, 192 pp, Quality PB, ISBN 1-879045-33-8 **$16.95**

The River of Light: *Spirituality, Judaism, Consciousness*
by Lawrence Kushner 6 x 9, 192 pp, Quality PB, ISBN 1-879045-03-6 **$14.95**

Spirituality & More

These Are the Words: *A Vocabulary of Jewish Spiritual Life*

by *Arthur Green*

What are the most essential ideas, concepts and terms that an educated person needs to know about Judaism? From *Adonai* (My Lord) to *zekhut* (merit), this enlightening and entertaining journey through Judaism teaches us the 149 core Hebrew words that constitute the basic vocabulary of Jewish spiritual life. 6 x 9, 304 pp, HC, ISBN 1-58023-024-5 **$21.95**

The Enneagram and Kabbalah: *Reading Your Soul*

by *Rabbi Howard A. Addison*

Combines two of the most powerful maps of consciousness known to humanity—The Tree of Life (the *Sefirot*) from the Jewish mystical tradition of *Kabbalah*, and the nine-pointed Enneagram—and shows how, together, they can provide a powerful tool for self-knowledge, critique, and transformation. 6 x 9, 176 pp, Quality PB, ISBN 1-58023-001-6 **$15.95**

Embracing the Covenant
Converts to Judaism Talk About Why & How

Ed. and with Intros. by *Rabbi Allan L. Berkowitz* and *Patti Moskovitz*

Through personal experiences of 20 converts to Judaism, this book illuminates reasons for converting, the quest for a satisfying spirituality, the appeal of the Jewish tradition and how conversion has changed lives—the convert's, and the lives of those close to them. 6 x 9, 192 pp, Quality PB, ISBN 1-879045-50-8 **$15.95**

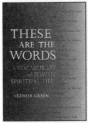 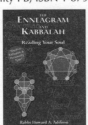 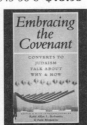 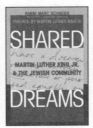 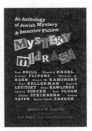

Shared Dreams: *Martin Luther King, Jr. and the Jewish Community*
by Rabbi Marc Schneier; Preface by Martin Luther King III
6 x 9, 240 pp, HC, ISBN 1-58023-062-8 **$24.95**

Mystery Midrash: *An Anthology of Jewish Mystery & Detective Fiction*
Ed. by Lawrence W. Raphael; Preface by Joel Siegel, ABC's *Good Morning America*
6 x 9, 304 pp, Quality PB, ISBN 1-58023-055-5 **$16.95**

The Jewish Gardening Cookbook: *Growing Plants & Cooking for Holidays & Festivals*
by Michael Brown 6 x 9, 224 pp, HC, Illus., ISBN 1-58023-004-0 **$21.95**

Wandering Stars: *An Anthology of Jewish Fantasy & Science Fiction* Ed. by Jack Dann; Intro. by Isaac Asimov 6 x 9, 272 pp, Quality PB, ISBN 1-58023-005-9 **$16.95**

More Wandering Stars
An Anthology of Outstanding Stories of Jewish Fantasy and Science Fiction
Ed. by Jack Dann; Intro. by Isaac Asimov 6 x 9, 192 pp, Quality PB, ISBN 1-58023-063-6 **$16.95**

A Heart of Wisdom: *Making the Jewish Journey from Midlife through the Elder Years*
Ed. by Susan Berrin; Foreword by Harold Kushner
6 x 9, 384 pp, Quality PB, ISBN 1-58023-051-2 **$18.95**; HC, ISBN 1-879045-73-7 **$24.95**

Sacred Intentions: *Daily Inspiration to Strengthen the Spirit, Based on Jewish Wisdom*
by Rabbi Kerry M. Olitzky and Rabbi Lori Forman
4½ x 6½, 448 pp, Quality PB, ISBN 1-58023-061-X **$15.95**

Theology/Philosophy

Torah of the Earth: *Exploring 4,000 Years of Ecology in Jewish Thought*
In 2 Volumes Ed. by *Rabbi Arthur Waskow*

Major new resource offering us an invaluable key to understanding the intersection of ecology and Judaism. Leading scholars provide us with a guided tour of ecological thought from four major Jewish viewpoints. Vol. 1: *Biblical Israel & Rabbinic Judaism*, 6 x 9, 272 pp, Quality PB, ISBN 1-58023-086-5 **$19.95**; Vol. 2: *Zionism & Eco-Judaism*, 6 x 9, 336 pp, Quality PB, ISBN 1-58023-087-3 **$19.95**

Broken Tablets: *Restoring the Ten Commandments and Ourselves*
Ed. by *Rabbi Rachel S. Mikva*; Intro. by *Rabbi Lawrence Kushner*;
Afterword by *Rabbi Arnold Jacob Wolf* **AWARD WINNER!**

Twelve outstanding spiritual leaders each share profound and personal thoughts about these biblical commands and why they have such a special hold on us.
6 x 9, 192 pp, HC, ISBN 1-58023-066-0 **$21.95**

Evolving Halakhah: *A Progressive Approach to Traditional Jewish Law*
by *Rabbi Dr. Moshe Zemer*

Innovative and provocative, this book affirms the system of traditional Jewish law, *halakhah*, as flexible enough to accommodate the changing realities of each generation. It shows that the traditional framework for understanding the Torah's commandments can be the living heart of Jewish life for all Jews. 6 x 9, 480 pp, HC, ISBN 1-58023-002-4 **$40.00**

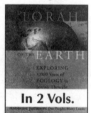 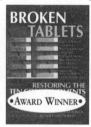 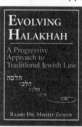 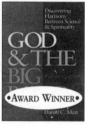 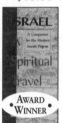

God & the Big Bang
Discovering Harmony Between Science & Spirituality **AWARD WINNER!**
by Daniel C. Matt
6 x 9, 216 pp, Quality PB, ISBN 1-879045-89-3 **$16.95**; HC, ISBN 1-879045-48-6 **$21.95**

Israel—A Spiritual Travel Guide **AWARD WINNER!**
A Companion for the Modern Jewish Pilgrim
by Rabbi Lawrence A. Hoffman 4¾ x 10, 256 pp, Quality PB, ISBN 1-879045-56-7 **$18.95**

Godwrestling—Round 2: *Ancient Wisdom, Future Paths* **AWARD WINNER!**
by Rabbi Arthur Waskow
6 x 9, 352 pp, Quality PB, ISBN 1-879045-72-9 **$18.95**; HC, ISBN 1-879045-45-1 **$23.95**

Ecology & the Jewish Spirit: *Where Nature & the Sacred Meet* Ed. and with Intros.
by Ellen Bernstein 6 x 9, 288 pp, Quality PB, ISBN 1-58023-082-2 **$16.95**;
HC, ISBN 1-879045-88-5 **$23.95**

Israel: *An Echo of Eternity* by Abraham Joshua Heschel; New Intro. by
Dr. Susannah Heschel 5½ x 8, 272 pp, Quality PB, ISBN 1-879045-70-2 **$18.95**

The Earth Is the Lord's: *The Inner World of the Jew in Eastern Europe*
by Abraham Joshua Heschel 5½ x 8, 112 pp, Quality PB, ISBN 1-879045-42-7 **$13.95**

A Passion for Truth: *Despair and Hope in Hasidism* by Abraham Joshua Heschel
5½ x 8, 352 pp, Quality PB, ISBN 1-879045-41-9 **$18.95**

Theology/Philosophy

A Heart of Many Rooms
Celebrating the Many Voices within Judaism
by *Dr. David Hartman* AWARD WINNER!

Named a *Publishers Weekly* "Best Book of the Year." Addresses the spiritual and theological questions that face all Jews and all people today. From the perspective of traditional Judaism, Hartman shows that commitment to both Jewish tradition and to pluralism can create understanding between people of different religious convictions.
6 x 9, 352 pp, HC, ISBN 1-58023-048-2 **$24.95**

A Living Covenant: *The Innovative Spirit in Traditional Judaism*
by *Dr. David Hartman* AWARD WINNER!

Winner, National Jewish Book Award. Hartman reveals a Judaism grounded in covenant—a relational framework—informed by the metaphor of marital love rather than that of parent-child dependency. 6 x 9, 368 pp, Quality PB, ISBN 1-58023-011-3 **$18.95**

The Death of Death: *Resurrection and Immortality in Jewish Thought*
by *Dr. Neil Gillman* AWARD WINNER!

Does death end life, or is it the passage from one stage of life to another? This National Jewish Book Award Finalist explores the original and compelling argument that Judaism, a religion often thought to pay little attention to the afterlife, not only offers us rich ideas on the subject—but delivers a deathblow to death itself. 6 x 9, 336 pp, Quality PB, ISBN 1-58023-081-4 **$18.95**; HC, ISBN 1-879045-61-3 **$23.95**

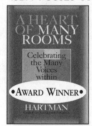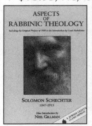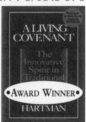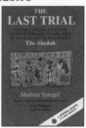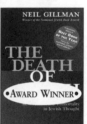

Aspects of Rabbinic Theology by Solomon Schechter; New Intro. by Dr. Neil Gillman
6 x 9, 448 pp, Quality PB, ISBN 1-879045-24-9 **$19.95**

The Last Trial: *On the Legends and Lore of the Command to Abraham to Offer Isaac as a Sacrifice* by Shalom Spiegel; New Intro. by Judah Goldin
6 x 9, 208 pp, Quality PB, ISBN 1-879045-29-X **$17.95**

Judaism and Modern Man: *An Interpretation of Jewish Religion* by Will Herberg; New Intro. by Dr. Neil Gillman 5½ x 8½, 336 pp, Quality PB, ISBN 1-879045-87-7 **$18.95**

Seeking the Path to Life AWARD WINNER!
Theological Meditations on God and the Nature of People, Love, Life and Death
by Rabbi Ira F. Stone
6 x 9, 160 pp, Quality PB, ISBN 1-879045-47-8 **$14.95**; HC, ISBN 1-879045-17-6 **$19.95**

The Spirit of Renewal: *Finding Faith after the Holocaust* AWARD WINNER!
by Rabbi Edward Feld
6 x 9, 224 pp, Quality PB, ISBN 1-879045-40-0 **$16.95**

Tormented Master: *The Life and Spiritual Quest of Rabbi Nahman of Bratslav*
by Dr. Arthur Green
6 x 9, 416 pp, Quality PB, ISBN 1-879045-11-7 **$18.95**

Your Word Is Fire: *The Hasidic Masters on Contemplative Prayer*
Ed. and Trans. with a New Introduction by Dr. Arthur Green and Dr. Barry W. Holtz
6 x 9, 160 pp, Quality PB, ISBN 1-879045-25-7 **$14.95**

Children's Spirituality

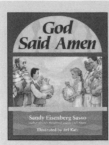

God Said Amen
by *Sandy Eisenberg Sasso*
Full-color illus. by *Avi Katz*

For ages 4 & up

MULTICULTURAL, NONDENOMINATIONAL, NONSECTARIAN

A warm and inspiring tale of two kingdoms: Midnight Kingdom is overflowing with water but has no oil to light its lamps; Desert Kingdom is blessed with oil but has no water to grow its gardens. The kingdoms' rulers ask God for help but are too stubborn to ask each other. It takes a minstrel, a pair of royal riding-birds and their young keepers, and a simple act of kindness to show that they need only reach out to each other to find God's answer to their prayers.

9 x 12, 32 pp, HC, Full-color illus., ISBN 1-58023-080-6 **$16.95**

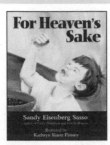

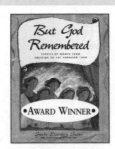

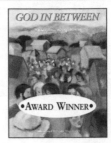

For Heaven's Sake
by *Sandy Eisenberg Sasso*; Full-color illus. by *Kathryn Kunz Finney*

For ages 4 & up

MULTICULTURAL, NONDENOMINATIONAL, NONSECTARIAN

Everyone talked about heaven: "Thank heavens." "Heaven forbid." "For heaven's sake, Isaiah." But no one would say what heaven was or how to find it. So Isaiah decides to find out, by seeking answers from many different people. "This book is a reminder of how well Sandy Sasso knows the minds of children. But it may surprise—and delight—readers to find how well she knows us grown-ups too." —*Maria Harris*, National Consultant in Religious Education, and author of *Teaching and Religious Imagination* 9 x 12, 32 pp, HC, Full-color illus., ISBN 1-58023-054-7 **$16.95**

But God Remembered: Stories of Women from Creation to the Promised Land
by *Sandy Eisenberg Sasso*; Full-color illus. by *Bethanne Andersen*

For ages 8 & up

NONDENOMINATIONAL, NONSECTARIAN

A fascinating collection of four different stories of women only briefly mentioned in biblical tradition and religious texts. Award-winning author Sasso vibrantly brings to life courageous and strong women from ancient tradition; all teach important values through their actions and faith. "Exquisite. . . . A book of beauty, strength and spirituality." —*Association of Bible Teachers* 9 x 12, 32 pp, HC, Full-color illus., ISBN 1-879045-43-5 **$16.95**

God in Between
by *Sandy Eisenberg Sasso*; Full-color illus. by *Sally Sweetland*

For ages 4 & up

MULTICULTURAL, NONDENOMINATIONAL, NONSECTARIAN

If you wanted to find God, where would you look? A magical, mythical tale that teaches that God can be found where we are: within all of us and the relationships between us. "This happy and wondrous book takes our children on a sweet and holy journey into God's presence." —*Rabbi Wayne Dosick, Ph.D.*, author of *Golden Rules* and *Soul Judaism*
9 x 12, 32 pp, HC, Full-color illus., ISBN 1-879045-86-9 **$16.95**

Children's Spirituality

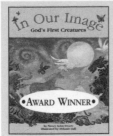

In Our Image
God's First Creatures
by *Nancy Sohn Swartz*
Full-color illus. by *Melanie Hall*

For ages 4 & up

NONDENOMINATIONAL, NONSECTARIAN

A playful new twist on the Creation story—from the perspective of the animals. Celebrates the interconnectedness of nature and the harmony of all living things. "The vibrantly colored illustrations nearly leap off the page in this delightful interpretation." —*School Library Journal*

"A message all children should hear, presented in words and pictures that children will find irresistible." —*Rabbi Harold Kushner*, author of *When Bad Things Happen to Good People*

9 x 12, 32 pp, HC, Full-color illus., ISBN 1-879045-99-0 **$16.95**

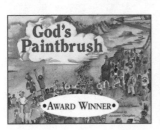

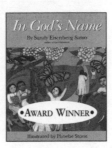

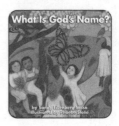

God's Paintbrush
by *Sandy Eisenberg Sasso*; Full-color illus. by *Annette Compton*

For ages 4 & up

MULTICULTURAL, NONDENOMINATIONAL, NONSECTARIAN

Invites children of all faiths and backgrounds to encounter God openly in their own lives. Wonderfully interactive; provides questions adult and child can explore together at the end of each episode. "An excellent way to honor the imaginative breadth and depth of the spiritual life of the young." —*Dr. Robert Coles*, Harvard University
11 x 8½, 32 pp, HC, Full-color illus., ISBN 1-879045-22-2 **$16.95**

Also available: **A Teacher's Guide: A Guide for Jewish & Christian Educators and Parents**
8½ x 11, 32 pp, PB, ISBN 1-879045-57-5 **$6.95**

God's Paintbrush Celebration Kit 9½ x 12, HC, Includes 5 sessions/40 full-color Activity Sheets and Teacher Folder with complete instructions, ISBN 1-58023-050-4 **$21.95**

In God's Name
by *Sandy Eisenberg Sasso*; Full-color illus. by *Phoebe Stone*

For ages 4 & up

MULTICULTURAL, NONDENOMINATIONAL, NONSECTARIAN

Like an ancient myth in its poetic text and vibrant illustrations, this award-winning modern fable about the search for God's name celebrates the diversity and, at the same time, the unity of all the people of the world. "What a lovely, healing book!" —*Madeleine L'Engle*
9 x 12, 32 pp, HC, Full-color illus., ISBN 1-879045-26-5 **$16.95**

What Is God's Name? (A Board Book)
An abridged board book version of the award-winning *In God's Name*.

For ages 0–4

5 x 5, 24 pp, Board, Full-color illus., ISBN 1-893361-10-1 **$7.95**

Children's Spirituality

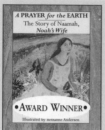

A Prayer for the Earth
The Story of Naamah, Noah's Wife
by *Sandy Eisenberg Sasso*
Full-color illus. by *Bethanne Andersen*

For ages 4 & up

NONDENOMINATIONAL, NONSECTARIAN

This new story, based on an ancient text, opens readers' religious imaginations to new ideas about the well-known story of the Flood. When God tells Noah to bring the animals of the world onto the ark, God also calls on Naamah, Noah's wife, to save each plant on Earth.

"A lovely tale. . . . Children of all ages should be drawn to this parable for our times."
—*Tomie dePaola*, artist/author of books for children

9 x 12, 32 pp, HC, Full-color illus., ISBN 1-879045-60-5 **$16.95**

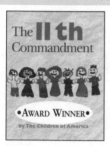

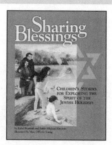

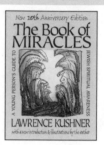

The 11th Commandment: Wisdom from Our Children
by The Children of America

For all ages

MULTICULTURAL, NONDENOMINATIONAL, NONSECTARIAN

"If there were an Eleventh Commandment, what would it be?" Children of many religious denominations across America answer this question—in their own drawings and words. "A rare book of spiritual celebration for all people, of all ages, for all time."—*Bookviews*
8 x 10, 48 pp, HC, Full-color illus., ISBN 1-879045-46-X **$16.95**

Sharing Blessings: Children's Stories for Exploring the Spirit of the Jewish Holidays
by *Rahel Musleah* and *Rabbi Michael Klayman*
Full-color illus. by *Mary O'Keefe Young*

For ages 6 & up

What is the spiritual message of each of the Jewish holidays? How do we teach it to our children? Many books tell children about the historical significance and customs of the holidays. Now, through engaging, creative stories about one family's preparation, *Sharing Blessings* explores ways to get into the *spirit* of 13 different holidays. "Lighthearted, and yet thorough—allows all Jewish parents (even those with very little Jewish education) to introduce the spirit of our cherished holiday traditions." —*Shari Lewis*, creator and star of PBS' *Lamb Chop's Play-Along*
8½ x 11, 64 pp, HC, Full-color illus., ISBN 1-879045-71-0 **$18.95**

The Book of Miracles
A Young Person's Guide to Jewish Spiritual Awareness
by *Lawrence Kushner*

For ages 9 & up

From the miracle at the Red Sea to the miracle of waking up this morning, this intriguing book introduces kids to a way of everyday spiritual thinking to last a lifetime. Kushner, whose award-winning books have brought spirituality to life for countless adults, now shows young people how to use Judaism as a foundation on which to build their lives. "A well-written, easy to understand, very lovely guide to Jewish spirituality. I recommend it to all teens as a good read." —*Kimberly Kirberger*, co-author, *Chicken Soup for the Teenage Soul* 6 x 9, 96 pp, HC, 2-color illus., ISBN 1-879045-78-8 **$16.95**

Life Cycle & Holidays

How to Be a Perfect Stranger, In 2 Volumes
A Guide to Etiquette in Other People's Religious Ceremonies
Ed. by *Stuart M. Matlins* & *Arthur J. Magida* **AWARD WINNER!**

What will happen? What do I do? What do I wear? What do I say? What should I avoid *doing, wearing, saying? What are their basic beliefs? Should I bring a gift?* In question-and-answer format, *How to Be a Perfect Stranger* explains the rituals and celebrations of America's major religions/denominations, helping an interested guest to feel comfortable, participate to the fullest extent possible, and avoid violating anyone's religious principles. It is not a guide to theology, nor is it presented from the perspective of any particular faith.

Vol. 1: *America's Largest Faiths,* 6 x 9, 432 pp, HC, ISBN 1-879045-39-7 **$24.95**
Vol. 2: *Other Faiths in America,* 6 x 9, 416 pp, HC, ISBN 1-879045-63-X **$24.95**

Putting God on the Guest List, 2nd Ed.
How to Reclaim the Spiritual Meaning of Your Child's Bar or Bat Mitzvah
by *Rabbi Jeffrey K. Salkin* **AWARD WINNER!**

The expanded, updated, revised edition of today's most influential book (over 60,000 copies in print) about finding core spiritual values in American Jewry's most misunderstood ceremony.
6 x 9, 224 pp, Quality PB, ISBN 1-879045-59-1 **$16.95**; HC, ISBN 1-879045-58-3 **$24.95**

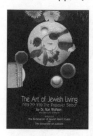 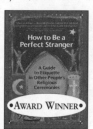 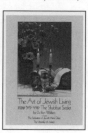 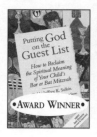 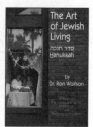

For Kids—Putting God on Your Guest List
How to Claim the Spiritual Meaning of Your Bar or Bat Mitzvah
by Rabbi Jeffrey K. Salkin 6 x 9, 144 pp, Quality PB, ISBN 1-58023-015-6 **$14.95**

Bar/Bat Mitzvah Basics
A Practical Family Guide to Coming of Age Together
Ed. by Cantor Helen Leneman 6 x 9, 240 pp, Quality PB, ISBN 1-879045-54-0 **$16.95**;
HC, ISBN 1-879045-51-6 **$24.95**

The New Jewish Baby Book AWARD WINNER!
Names, Ceremonies, & Customs—A Guide for Today's Families
by Anita Diamant 6 x 9, 336 pp, Quality PB, ISBN 1-879045-28-1 **$16.95**

Hanukkah: The Art of Jewish Living
by Dr. Ron Wolfson 7 x 9, 192 pp, Quality PB, Illus., ISBN 1-879045-97-4 **$16.95**

The Shabbat Seder: The Art of Jewish Living
by Dr. Ron Wolfson 7 x 9, 272 pp, Quality PB, Illus., ISBN 1-879045-90-7 **$16.95**
Also available are these helpful companions to *The Shabbat Seder*: Booklet of the Blessings and Songs, ISBN 1-879045-91-5 **$5.00**; Audiocassette of the Blessings, DN03 **$6.00**; Teacher's Guide, ISBN 1-879045-92-3 **$4.95**

The Passover Seder: The Art of Jewish Living
by Dr. Ron Wolfson 7 x 9, 352 pp, Quality PB, Illus., ISBN 1-879045-93-1 **$16.95**
Also available are these helpful companions to *The Passover Seder*: Passover Workbook, ISBN 1-879045-94-X **$6.95**; Audiocassette of the Blessings, DN04 **$6.00**; Teacher's Guide, ISBN 1-879045-95-8 **$4.95**

Life Cycle

Jewish Paths toward Healing and Wholeness
A Personal Guide to Dealing with Suffering
by *Rabbi Kerry M. Olitzky*; Foreword by *Debbie Friedman*

"Why me?" Why do we suffer? How can we heal? Grounded in the spiritual traditions of Judaism, this book provides healing rituals, psalms and prayers that help readers initiate a dialogue with God, to guide them along the complicated path of healing and wholeness.
6 x 9, 192 pp, Quality PB, ISBN 1-58023-068-7 **$15.95**

Mourning & Mitzvah: *A Guided Journal for Walking the Mourner's Path through Grief to Healing*
by *Anne Brener*, L.C.S.W.; Foreword by *Rabbi Jack Riemer*; Intro. by *Rabbi William Cutter*

For those who mourn a death, for those who would help them, for those who face a loss of any kind, Brener teaches us the power and strength available to us in the fully experienced mourning process. 7½ x 9, 288 pp, Quality PB, ISBN 1-879045-23-0 **$19.95**

Tears of Sorrow, Seeds of Hope
A Jewish Spiritual Companion for Infertility and Pregnancy Loss
by *Rabbi Nina Beth Cardin*

A spiritual companion that enables us to mourn infertility, a lost pregnancy, or a stillbirth within the prayers, rituals, and meditations of Judaism. By drawing on the texts of tradition, it creates readings and rites of mourning, and through them provides a wellspring of compassion, solace—and hope. 6 x 9, 192 pp, HC, ISBN 1-58023-017-2 **$19.95**

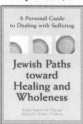 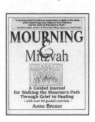 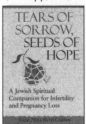 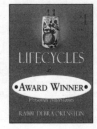 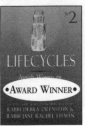

Lifecycles
V. 1: *Jewish Women on Life Passages & Personal Milestones* AWARD WINNER!
Ed. and with Intros. by Rabbi Debra Orenstein
V. 2: *Jewish Women on Biblical Themes in Contemporary Life* AWARD WINNER!
Ed. and with Intros. by Rabbi Debra Orenstein and Rabbi Jane Rachel Litman
V. 1: 6 x 9, 480 pp, Quality PB, ISBN 1-58023-018-0 **$19.95**; HC, ISBN 1-879045-14-1 **$24.95**
V. 2: 6 x 9, 464 pp, Quality PB, ISBN 1-58023-019-9 **$19.95**; HC, ISBN 1-879045-15-X **$24.95**

Grief in Our Seasons: *A Mourner's Kaddish Companion*
by Rabbi Kerry M. Olitzky 4½ x 6½, 448 pp, Quality PB, ISBN 1-879045-55-9 **$15.95**

A Time to Mourn, A Time to Comfort: *A Guide to Jewish Bereavement and Comfort*
by Dr. Ron Wolfson 7 x 9, 336 pp, Quality PB, ISBN 1-879045-96-6 **$16.95**

When a Grandparent Dies
A Kid's Own Remembering Workbook for Dealing with Shiva and the Year Beyond
by Nechama Liss-Levinson, Ph.D.
8 x 10, 48 pp, HC, Illus., 2-color text, ISBN 1-879045-44-3 **$15.95**

So That Your Values Live On: *Ethical Wills & How to Prepare Them*
Ed. by Rabbi Jack Riemer & Professor Nathaniel Stampfer
6 x 9, 272 pp, Quality PB, ISBN 1-879045-34-6 **$17.95**